Lars Holm Tjessem

Application of Bacteriophages in Clinical Medicine

AF190961

Lars Holm Tjessem

Application of Bacteriophages in Clinical Medicine

Solution to Antibiotic Resistance?

Reihe Realwissenschaften

Imprint

Any brand names and product names mentioned in this book are subject to trademark, brand or patent protection and are trademarks or registered trademarks of their respective holders. The use of brand names, product names, common names, trade names, product descriptions etc. even without a particular marking in this work is in no way to be construed to mean that such names may be regarded as unrestricted in respect of trademark and brand protection legislation and could thus be used by anyone.

Cover image: www.ingimage.com

Publisher:
AV Akademikerverlag
is a trademark of
Dodo Books Indian Ocean Ltd. and OmniScriptum S.R.L publishing group

120 High Road, East Finchley, London, N2 9ED, United Kingdom
Str. Armeneasca 28/1, office 1, Chisinau MD-2012, Republic of Moldova, Europe
Managing Directors: Ieva Konstantinova, Victoria Ursu
info@omniscriptum.com

Printed at: see last page
ISBN: 978-3-639-80626-7

1   Table of Contents

2 Acknowledgements

I would like to thank my tutor and supervisor Professor Wolfgang M. Prodinger for his invaluable input, advice, and guidance throughout the process of writing this thesis. Thank you for letting me choose my own research topic, for believing in me, and for the time you have invested in this project. I will remember our meetings and discussions, and bring with me your advice and everything you have taught me.

I would also like to thank my wonderful family for all your support and love. My dear Lea, Linde, and Amalie, thank you for letting me spend so much time on this thesis. Thank you for your support, encouragement, and the inspiration you have given me, and most of all thank you for making me laugh every day. I am also forever grateful for the everlasting support from my family in Norway.

To all of you who have helped me in any way, and especially my young girls, I could not have done this without you. This work is dedicated to all of you.

3 Zusammenfassung (in German)

Die Verwendung von Bakteriophagen zur Therapie einer bakteriellen Infektion, die Phagentherapie, wird oft als ein möglicher Ausweg aus den Schwierigkeiten durch die Zunehmende Antibiotikaresistenz gesehen. In dieser Arbeit werden die wichtigsten Hindernisse für die Phagentherapie sowie die Machbarkeit einer echten Therapieoption in Europa und Nordamerika analysiert und diskutiert. Frühere Arbeiten haben die Geschichte und das Potenzial der Phagentherapie sowie die großen Probleme und Herausforderungen diskutiert, es gibt jedoch keine umfassende Machbarkeitsstudie zu dem Thema. Diese Arbeit wurde als systematische Literaturanalyse durchgeführt.

Der Verfasser Stellt fest, dass in der aktuellen juristischen und pharmakoökonomischen Situation in Europa und Nordamerika die Phagentherapie auf der Basis natürlicher Bakteriophagen noch nicht als machbare Alternative zu Antibiotika berücksichtigt werden kann. Sinnvolle und nachhaltigen Phagentherapie kann nur im Rahmen eines spezifischen Gesetz, die die Dynamik des Bakteriophagen Arzneimittels und das Eigentum der Investoren berücksichtigen entwickelt werden. Die Situation ist jedoch anders für Produkte die aus Bakteriophagen stammen, wie Endolysine und konstruierte Wirkstoffabgabesystem, die eine viel bessere Aussicht haben in neue antimikrobielle Mittel entwickelt zu werden.

4 Abstract

The use of bacteriophages to treat bacterial infection, *i.e.*, phage therapy, is often seen as one of the possible remedies for the current antibiotic resistance crisis. In this thesis, the major hindrances to phage therapy as well as its feasibility as a real therapeutic option in Europe and North America are explored and discussed. Previous work has discussed the history and potential of phage therapy, as well as its major problems and challenges. There is however to date no comprehensive feasibility study on the topic. This thesis has been undertaken as a systematic literature review.

The author finds that under the current regulatory and pharmacoeconomical situation in Europe and North America, phage therapy based on natural bacteriophages cannot be considered as a feasible alternative to antibiotics. Sensible and sustainable phage therapy can only be developed under a specific legal framework that take into account the dynamics of bacteriophage pharmaceuticals and protects the property of investors. The situation is, however, different for products derived from bacteriophages, such as phage lysins and engineered drug-delivery systems, which face a much brighter prospect to be developed into novel antimicrobial agents.

5 Introduction

Bacterial infections in humans range from small local infections that mostly cause nuisance or perhaps no symptoms at all, to systemic, life-threatening, and disabling illness. These have been a danger to humans for as long as we have existed, and will undoubtedly continue to haunt us for the remainder of our time. We have, however, also always tried to combat and treat these infections, first using substances found in nature, and later synthetic drugs (1). For the last 70 years, we have had great help from antibiotics in this fight. In the same time-span we have also been able to observe ongoing evolution, when we witnessed the development of antibiotic resistant bacteria (2). As we are on the verge of losing our primary weapon against bacteria it becomes clear that we need to investigate other treatment options (3,4).

In his Nobel lecture, Sir Alexander Fleming warned the scientific community about resistance to antibiotics. Shortly thereafter, the first reports of staphylococcal resistance to penicillin started to emerge, thus making it clear that bacterial resistance to antibiotics is an Darwinian consequence to antibiotic use (2). This was nevertheless not perceived as troublesome situation because new classes of antibiotics continued to be developed in the glory days of the 1950s (ref. (5)). However, the antibiotic development pipeline has since run dry, well-illustrated by the fact that only four new classes of antibiotics have been discovered since 1960 (ref. (6)).

Concerns about antibiotic resistance have intensified in the last two decades as an increasing number of multidrug resistant, and even pan-resistant bacteria emerge (2). Although efforts have been taken to reduce the consumption of antibiotics and alleviate the situation, treatment-resistant bacterial infections still claim thousands of lives yearly, and confer high costs to the health care systems (3,6). Researchers also agree that the problem of antibiotic resistance will not vanish by simply reducing the amount of antibiotics used, and that there is a justified and urgent need to develop new classes of antibiotics and other novel antimicrobial drugs (2,3,5–7).

During the last decade extensive research, mainly driven by the academic community, into novel treatment options for bacterial infections have yielded many possibilities, but none that are found to have the full potential to replace antibiotics (7). Research into antimicrobial peptides, therapeutic antibodies, vaccines, and potentiators of currently used antibiotics are ongoing, but currently years from yielding any products for market placement. Another, treatment option, which cannot be considered as novel, is the use of bacterial viruses, bacteriophages, for treatment of infections. Also known as phage therapy, this concept have been practiced in certain areas of the world for almost 90 years. This thesis will investigate phage therapy as a treatment alternative to antibiotics, and discuss the feasibility of a possible reintroduction of phage therapy in Europe and North America.

6   Scope of Thesis

This thesis, dealing with the antimicrobial use of bacteriophages, finds it foundation in the current situation of increasing antibiotic resistance of pathogens. The precise aim is to explore and identify the main obstacles and challenges that antimicrobial bacteriophage therapy is facing and to determine, whether phage therapy is one feasible way out of the antibiotic resistance crisis. With the aim of answering this question in a comprehensive manner, a detailed study of the historical use of therapeutic bacteriophages is required, together with an investigation and discussion of current clinical and legal aspects of phage therapy.

To this end, this study is designed as a systematic literature review with defined search strategy, inclusion and exclusion criteria, and data extraction method.

7 Methodology

The development of an appropriate study design for this project went through several phases. After selection of the research topic and question, a preliminary search of available literature was performed. This search revealed that the majority of available studies on this subject are reviews, with relatively few qualitative or quantitative studies. With this information, a study protocol was written with the aim of creating a framework for a systematic literature review. The main topics and steps in the study protocol are outlined in the sections below.

7.1 Review Question

The review question chosen for this thesis is:

> *"Which impediments need to be surmounted for antimicrobial bacteriophage therapy to be accepted and developed as a feasible alternative to conventional antibiotics?"*

In order to identify these obstacles, it will in the course of this project be necessary to elaborate on the history of bacteriophages, their mechanism of action, documented use and trials, and their possible medical applications against bacterial infections.

7.2 Search Strategy

The search strategy was developed as a two-step process where an electronic search string was first employed. The results of this search were evaluated against the inclusion and exclusion criteria, whereby the reference section of the included papers were hand searched for additional literature.

The following search string was employed at Web of Science, Medline, Current Content Connect, EMBASE, Biological Abstracts, and ISI Highly Cited.

- *(bacteriophage OR phage therapy) AND (antibiotics OR antibiotic resistance OR anti infectious OR history OR pharmacokinetic OR immunological response) AND (therapy OR treatment OR alternative treatment OR clinical trial) NOT (phage display OR surveillance) AND (Humans[Mesh] AND (German[lang] OR Swedish[lang] OR Danish[lang] OR English[lang] OR Norwegian[lang]))*

7.3 Literature Selection Criteria and Procedure

The following inclusion and exclusion criteria were used to evaluate the results from the search process (table 1). Only studies that conformed to these criteria were eligible for inclusion, and went on to the coding process.

Table 1 - Inclusion and Exclusion Criteria

	Inclusion criteria	Exclusion criteria
Population or focus	- Anti infectious therapy - Human medicine - Bacteriophage virology - History and documented use of phage therapy - Legal framework with regard to phage application - Immunological response	- Phage display - Veterinary medicine - Agricultural application - Other than anti-infectious application - Species-specific in vitro experiments
Outcome	All outcomes	
Study design	All other	Editorials, biological patents, interviews, conference proceedings.
Publication date	All	
Publication language	English German Norwegian Swedish Danish	All other

The studies found in the search were evaluated against these criteria in several steps.

1. Initial screening:
   - The titles of all studies were first evaluated. Publications clearly irrelevant to this project were excluded.

2. Assessing abstracts:
   - The abstracts of the remaining publications were assessed against the inclusion and exclusion criteria.

3. Assessing full text articles:
   - All articles that were included on the basis of their abstract (and articles without abstract) were retrieved in full text.

[10]

- All full-text articles were thoroughly examined and evaluated against the inclusion and exclusion criteria.
- All full-text publications that passed the final round of assessment were logged in the Mendeley Reference and Project Manager software, and proceeded to the coding and data extraction step.

7.4 Coding and Data Extraction

With the purpose of grouping the included studies, as well as for standardising the data extracted from them, all articles were coded using an adapted coding sheet. The coding sheet was designed to extract both objective data about each study, as well as data from the author's findings and conclusions. See the appendix of this thesis for an example of the coding sheet.

The coding sheet was piloted by the author and his supervisor (*i.e.*, "the reviewers") for completeness and suitability. Each reviewer coded the same four full-text publications selected from the included publications. The reviewers jointly discussed their coding of the publications and modified the coding sheet according to their findings. Then, both reviewers coded a set of 4 new publications in order to finalize the coding sheet for use for the coding of the remaining articles.

During the coding the studies were also assigned thematic groups and labelled accordingly in the Mendeley software. This grouping served as tool for arranging the studies by topic, before synthesis of the review, and is presented in the appendix of this thesis.

7.5 Synthesis of Review

After the coding of all included studies, the extracted data was compiled into the findings presented in the results section below. Since the data that had been extracted according to the pre-determined explicit method showed great variety based on research design and presentation, the author chose to present his findings using narrative writing.

8 Results

The two-step search process yielded in total 74 studies that were eligible for inclusion to this thesis (Fig. 1). Literature reviews accounted for 66 % of the included studies, with the remainder being case studies, clinical trials, laboratory studies, books, and laws (Fig. 2). The majority of the studies were published from 2003 and onwards, signalling a renewed interest in phage therapy in the last decade. A graph detailing the time of publication of included articles is presented in the appendix.

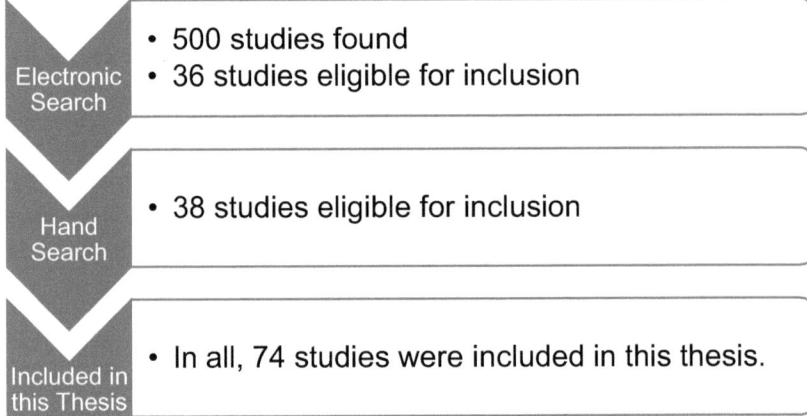

Figure 1 - Results of the Search Process

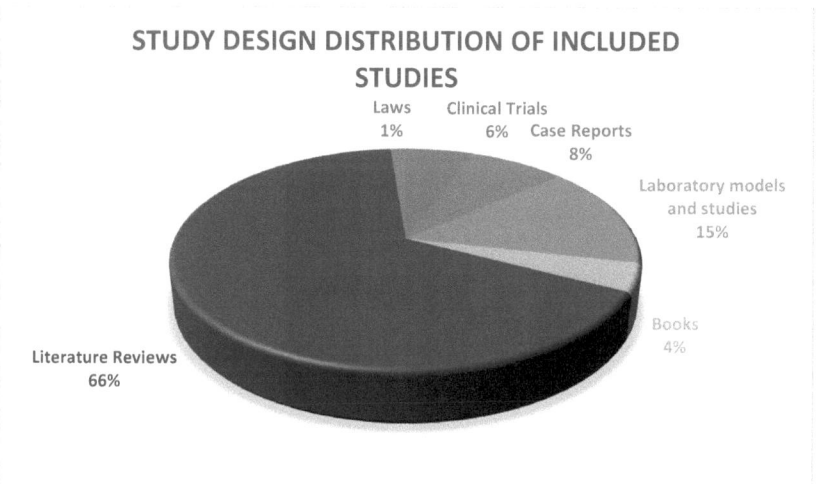

Figure 2 - Study design distribution of included studies.

In the following sections, the result of the extracted data is presented. Starting with an introduction to what phage therapy really is and how it works, this chapter follows a chronological order to bring the reader through the history of phage therapy up to the current situation where the review question is discussed.

8.1 Phage Therapy

Bacteriophages are the viruses of bacteria, and perhaps the most abundant life-form on earth (8). Bacteriophage therapy, or simply phage therapy, is the use of bacteriophages to control and treat human infections. The principals of phage therapy are, and have been since its conception, to introduce bacteriophages to the disease causing bacterial flora. The phages then infect the bacteria and convert them into factories for producing new phages (Fig. 3). Once the bacterial machinery is hijacked in this manner, the bacteria are actually considered dead.

However, each bacterium will continue to produce 100 - 300 new virions until lysis occurs. The new phages are then released, and able to attach to uninfected bacteria and repeat the infectious cycle. Through this process, the bacteriophages are able, under the right conditions, to increase in number *in vivo* and effectively kill all pathogenic bacteria. Due to the fact that bacteriophages exhibit a narrow host-range, one can ensure through careful selection of therapeutic phages, that the physiological flora of the patient remains untouched (9,10).

The bacteriophages are usually given as a cocktail, containing several different phages, or as a solution containing a single type of phage, so called adapted phage, that is proven to be lytic and selected against bacterial strains isolated from the individual patient (11).

There are numerous factors with respect to the biology of bacteriophages, their pharmacological properties, clinical application, immunological response, and safety involved in phage therapy. These factors will be described in detail in the chapters that follows.

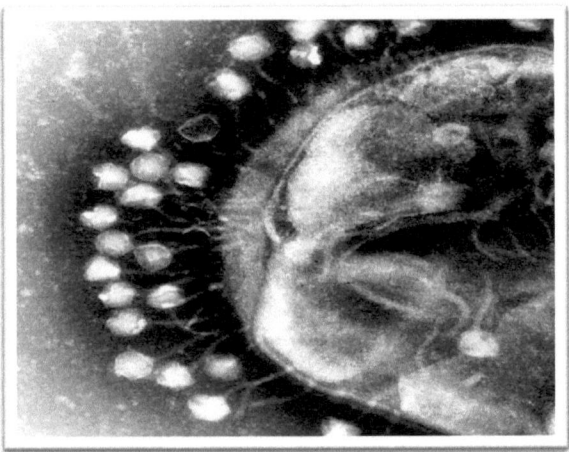

Figure 3 - Coliphage T1 attached to a bacterium. Source: Wikimedia Commons.

8.2 The History of Phage Therapy

The history of phage therapy is full of enthusiasm, over-exaggeration, disappointment, optimism, promise, and potential (Fig. 4). In order to understand the potential and obstacles of using bacteriophages to treat human bacterial infections, it is important to learn about the use of bacteriophages in the past and the results obtained.

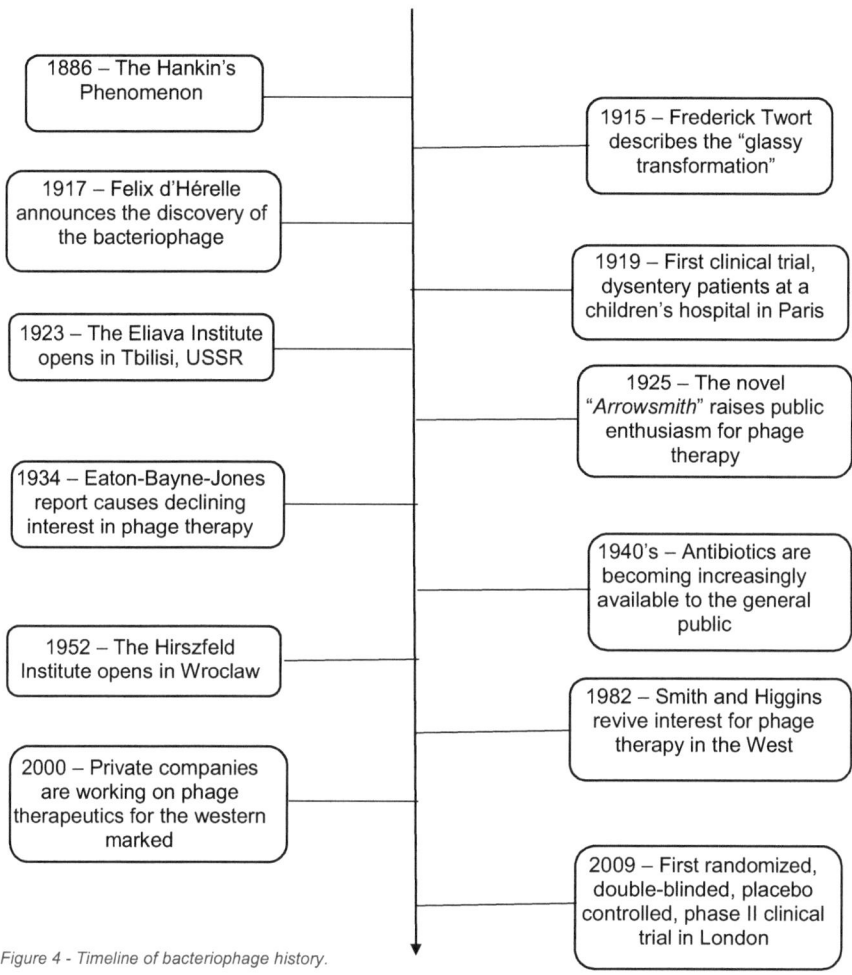

Figure 4 - Timeline of bacteriophage history.

The following text boxes appear in the timeline:

1886 – The Hankin's Phenomenon

1915 – Frederick Twort describes the "glassy transformation"

1917 – Felix d'Hérelle announces the discovery of the bacteriophage

1919 – First clinical trial, dysentery patients at a children's hospital in Paris

1923 – The Eliava Institute opens in Tbilisi, USSR

1925 – The novel "*Arrowsmith*" raises public enthusiasm for phage therapy

1934 – Eaton-Bayne-Jones report causes declining interest in phage therapy

1940's – Antibiotics are becoming increasingly available to the general public

1952 – The Hirszfeld Institute opens in Wroclaw

1982 – Smith and Higgins revive interest for phage therapy in the West

2000 – Private companies are working on phage therapeutics for the western marked

2009 – First randomized, double-blinded, placebo controlled, phase II clinical trial in London

8.2.1 The Discovery of Bacteriophages

The question of who discovered bacteriophages is the subject to much debate. The British bacteriologist Ernest Hankin described the "Hankin's phenomenon" when he in 1886 reported the antibacterial activity in the Ganges and Jumna rivers in India (12). Many authors interpret this observation as a reference to bacteriophage activity, however not all, and some have even gone to considerable length to prove that the "Hankin's phenomenon" must be caused by some other agent (11–13). Even though the literature also offers numerous other historic phage references none of these amounted to any real evidence of the causative agent (10,14).

[15]

In 1915, the British medical doctor and bacteriologist Frederick Twort published an article in *The Lancet* where he described the minute "glassy transformation" or clear zone of lysis of colonies of *Staphylococcus* on agar plates (15). He further described how he filtered the affected colonies and introduced the filtrate onto other colonies of *Staphylococcus*, thereby creating new clear zones. He therefore termed this phenomenon as an "acute infectious disease" of the bacteria, and postulated that it might be, among other things, caused by a virus. Regrettably, Twort was unable to continue his research due to financial concerns because of World War 1.

Two years later, the French-Canadian microbiologist Félix d`Hérelle, working at the Pasteur Institute in Paris, published his article *"About an invisible microbe antagonistic to dysentery bacilli"* (12). In this article, published in the meeting proceedings from a meeting of the Academy of Sciences in September 1917, d`Hérelle described how he during an outbreak of dysentery among French soldiers observed clear zones or *plaques* on agar medium cultivated with faecal samples from the diseased (16). This observation, almost identical to that of Twort two years earlier led d`Hérelle to conclude that a virus parasitic of bacteria was the causative agent. With this, he coined the term "bacteriophage" (14). D`Hérelle observed that there was a correlation between the number of plaque counts on agar medium and the recovery from dysentery, and derived from this that bacteriophages were "exogenous agents of immunity" (12).

D`Hérelle maintained that his discovery was distinct from that of Twort, and considered himself the discoverer of bacteriophages. This has however been the subject to much dispute and discussion, while some scientists accept the independent discovery of Twort and d`Hérelle others cite Twort as the first discoverer and state that d`Hérelle extended Twort´s research (11,12).

The announcement of the discovery of the bacteriophage was not widely accepted at the time (11). A strong scientific posse, led by Jules Bordet, challenged the view that the causative agent in question was a virus. They believed that the "Twort - d`Hérelle phenomenon" was a result of enzymatic activity or other soluble substance. This controversy continued throughout the 1920s and 1930s, and ended only with the visualization of bacteriophages by electron microscopy in 1942 (ref. (12)).

8.2.2 Early studies and commercialization

D`Hérelle very soon understood the potential of bacteriophage for treatment of bacterial infections. What is most likely the first study in phage therapy was conducted by d`Hérelle at a children's hospital in Paris in 1919. D`Hérelle used a phage preparation, containing phages obtained from stool samples of soldiers with dysentery, to treat several children with severe dysentery (9). Before the study commenced, d`Hérelle and the hospital's Chief of Paediatrics, Professor Victor-Henri Hutinel, ingested the phage preparation in order to confirm its safety. D`Hérelle treated four patients with severe dysentery with a single dose of bacteriophages, noting that all four recovered fully within a few days (11). Due to the fact that d`Hérelle did not publish his findings until a few years after, the first published use of phage therapy in human infections came from Richard Bruynoghe and Joseph Maisin in 1921 (14).

Bruynoghe and Maisin, working in Belgium, reported in their article the reduction in swelling, pain and fever in six patients with cutaneous boils, 48 hours after injecting a phage preparation into the base of the boils (9). Encouraged by these early positive results, and other published phage therapy studies, d`Hérelle continued to undertake extensive studies into clinical application of bacteriophages, especially directed towards treatment of typhoid fever and cholera, as well as refining his method of preparation of therapeutic bacteriophages (9,11).

At the same time d`Hérelle took steps to commercialise bacteriophage preparations for infectious disease through the French company *Societé Française de Tenitures Inoffensives pour Cheveux*, now L'Oreal (12). They produced five different phage cocktails, where each cocktail contained several different bacteriophages sensitive to different pathogenic bacteria, targeting intestinal, nasal, purulent and staphylococcal infections (11).

Bacteriophage therapy caught the public eye and gained popularity through the 1925 novel *Arrowsmith*, written by Sinclair Lewis. This book tells the story of a young physician who attempts to cure plague with bacteriophages (12). Then, during the 1920s and 1930s pharmaceutical companies in the western world started to produce and distribute their own bacteriophage products, including such companies as Eli Lilly (US), Antipol (Germany) and Medico-Biological Laboratories (UK) (17).

8.2.3 Downfall

Regardless of all the optimism, commercial products and studies in favour of phage therapy, interest in using bacteriophages to treat human infections slowly vanished in the western world throughout the 1930s and 1940s (9). The reasons behind this demise is often, and also partly correct, attributed to the advent of antibiotics (12,18). The fact is that there were problems that are more complex and unresolved issues and questions, some even valid today, that also contributed greatly to the marginalization of bacteriophage therapy in the western world. More specifically, the problems of exaggerated claims, insufficient knowledge and manufacturing techniques, failure to establish scientific proof and a whole range of highly weighted negative reviews were instrumental in asphyxiating the phage therapy interest (table 2) (ref.(11,19)).

Table 2 - The most frequently cited problems with early phage therapy, as presented by Sulakvelidze (11).

Problem	Comments	Solution
Narrow host range of phages	Early phage treatment often yielded negative results due to failure to select phages lytic for the target bacteria.	Use of phage cocktails with phages effective on the majority of strains of the target bacteria, or use of adapted phages.
Insufficient purity of phage preparations	Early production techniques yielded only crude lysates which contained dangerous and pathogenic contaminants.	Modern production techniques as high speed centrifugation and EndoTrap®, allows for phage preparations of high purity.(20)
Poor stability and viability of phage preparations	Many of the early preparations received heat treatment and various additives that inactivated the phages.	Modern production techniques removes the need for heating and titer-lowering additives.
Lack of knowledge about the biology of bacteriophages	Lack of knowledge led investigators to choose lysogenic phages instead of lytic ones.	Cautious selection of lytic phages.
Exaggerated claims of effectiveness	Some cocktails were marketed as effective against viral infections.	Phage preparations must be developed with proper scientific documentation about their effectiveness.
Failure to establish scientific proof of efficacy.	Most clinical studies on phage therapy do not meet the standards of double blind, placebo controlled trials.	All new clinical trials must adhere to GCP/GLP and meet the standards of controlled trials, in order to determine a solid scientific base.

During the early days of phage therapy the results form poorly controlled trials and mass media created a hype of enthusiasm. As with any new technology or fashion, commercial players sought to profit on phage therapy as described in the chapter above. Some of these commercial products came with widely exaggerated claims. An example of this is the product *Enterophagos,* which was allegedly effective against many conditions, including viral infections such as herpes or generalized conditions such as urticaria and eczema (19). It is not known whether or not this overstatement of efficacy came from insufficient knowledge about microbiology and infectious diseases, or if it was just an immoral sales pitch. Whatever the reason, the fact remains that this type of misleading marketing was an influential factor in bringing about an overall scepticism against phage therapy among the general population.

Throughout the first two decades of phage therapy, insufficient knowledge about bacteriophages, their biology and isolation, further contributed to bad results and inability to live up to its high expectations. This lack of knowledge led to in some places that hygiene and vaccines against cholera were replaced by bacteriophages introduced to the village well, with the obvious terrible results (19). Furthermore, early preparations of therapeutic bacteriophages were often crude lysates of host bacteria, containing many contaminants such as endotoxins, capable of inducing severe side effects and reduced the effect of the phages (11). In addition, little work was done to select active, strain-specific phages and very little was known about the virulence of bacteria. The result was that many of the commercially available phage preparations had no or little activity titers to the field strain in question (9,19). Even though a few well-performed studies in the 1930s and 1940s showed that therapeutic effect of bacteriophages was possible under controlled conditions, damage was already done to the paradigm of phage therapy (19).

Moreover, one of the most central elements that have led to doubt and hesitation concerning phage therapy, is the almost complete lack of appropriately conducted, placebo-controlled studies. This has been evident since the very first trials of phage therapy, and is still a major issue today (11). Uncontrolled studies, in combination with the already described problems of insufficient knowledge and overstated claims of efficacy, further fuelled the controversy of phage therapy in the scientific community.

As a response to this debate and disagreement on phage therapy, the American Medical Association commissioned a full review of all available literature on phage therapy (11). This resulted in the 1934 Eaton-Bayne-Jones report which reviewed more than 100 studies on bacteriophage therapy (21). Overall, a negative review with respect to phage therapy, the authors also stated that evidence indicated that the bacteriophage is not a virus, but rather an enzyme. This report had a strong negative impact on the attitude of agencies funding bacteriophage research. Further negative reviews followed throughout the 1940s which together with the Eaton-Bayne-Jones report effectively stopped all major studies of phage therapy in western academic societies (9,11).

In post-war Europe and North-America, antibiotics became generally available to the common man which further decimated interest in phage therapy (17). The final nail in the coffin for bacteriophage therapy in the West came in 1959, when the World Health Organization came to the conclusion that, with the success of tetracycline therapy there was no reason for research into bacteriophage therapy to continue (19).

8.2.4 Continued use and research

With phage therapy effectively dead in the mainstream academic societies in the West by 1950, research, development and use of phage therapy continued behind the iron curtain in the Soviet Union and Eastern Europe.

For decades, these centres have continued to explore, develop and apply bacteriophages as a therapeutic option (22). However, due to the geopolitical situation from the 1940s until the beginning of the 1990s, the scientific studies from these centres in the Soviet Union and Eastern Europe were not readily published in internationally available journals. This is in part due to the fact that phage therapy research was considered a state secret in the Soviet Union (9). Therefore, it is only in the last decade that all this accumulated knowledge and lessons learned are becoming available to the scientific community in the rest of the world (3).

In the following chapters, the story of this continued research and use will be told. In addition to focusing on the major phage therapy centres in Georgia and Poland, the continued use by small groups of practitioners in France and elsewhere in the West will also be discussed.

8.2.5   The Soviet Union and Georgia

Since the very beginning of the phage therapy era, practitioners and scientists have found a "safe" home in the Soviet Union, and in today's successor states Russia and Georgia. Bacteriophage therapy has become standard medical care in these countries, and much is to be learned from their experience. This chapter will first rekindle the history and status of the Eliava Institute in Tbilisi, Georgia, and then review the clinical studies, trials, and work done in the Soviet Union as a whole.

8.2.5.1   The Eliava Institute

The George Eliava Institute opened its doors in 1923 in the Georgian capital Tbilisi. Its founder and first director was George Eliava who had worked at the Pasteur Institute in Paris together with Felix d'Hérelle from 1919 to 1921. Upon returning from Paris, he brought with him laboratory equipment worth 100,000 Francs, as a gift from the Pasteur Institute (14). Eliava and d'Hérelle continued to work closely together, and shared the vision of making Eliava's microbiology institute into a world centre of bacteriophage research and therapy. With the blessing from the General Secretary of the Communist Party of the Soviet Union, Joseph Stalin, the centre became a reality (23). However, George Eliava, a colourful figure, was arrested in 1937 and executed without a trail as a "people's enemy" for being in intellectual opposition to Lavrenti Beria, the chief of the secret police (14). Stunned and decapitated, the Eliava Institute managed to survive and continued to develop its centre into a large facility, employing more than 1200 people, building an extensive phage collection, and also establishing production facilities elsewhere in the Soviet Union (9,14).

The Eliava Institute has focused their primary efforts on producing therapeutic phage cocktails, where each cocktail encompasses many different phages targeting a certain group of pathogenic bacteria. Their secondary efforts have focused on production of vaccines, antisera and individualized treatment (23).

The Eliava Institute soon became a corner stone in the Soviet health system, and received bacterial samples from all over the Soviet Union for use in developing and adjusting phage cocktails. At the height of its prominence in the 1980s the Institute produced more than 2 metric tons of phage products, each week (23). These phage products were mainly tablets and solutions targeting gastrointestinal and wound infections. The main consumer of these products was the Red Army, who depended heavily on these medications and received 80 % of the production, the rest being available to the public (9). With its unique position as a supplier to the military and as a centre of competence, the research and production was regarded as a military secret, thereby prohibiting publication of much of its work (23).

With the fragmentation of the Soviet Union in the early 1990s, the Institute lost its funding source and biggest consumer, with the result that most of its production facilities were privatized and put to other uses. Even though the Eliava Institute suffered severe economic hardship during the early years of Georgia's regained independence, it enjoyed strong political support which together with significant private investments helped the Institute survive (23).

Through the investment from mainly Georgian medical personnel and international institutions, the Institute is today thriving and collaborating with many major research institutions around the world. The Eliava Institute have in the recently founded several spin-off companies, such as JSC Biochimpharm and Eliava Biopreparations Ltd, who produce and distribute prophylactic and therapeutic phage products. The Eliava Phage Therapy Centre, a day clinic, opened its doors in 2010, and renders its services to both local and foreign patients (14,23).

The Eliava Institute, through its spin-off companies and collaborators, produces and markets several prophylactic and therapeutic phage cocktails, some of them available to the public in Russia and Georgia without prescription. Two of these products are generically named *pyophage and intestiphage*. These are phage cocktails, which contains a battery of different phages targeting problematic bacteria. The licensed products are required by law to be tested against an extensive array of emerging problematic strains and, if necessary, retested and updated every six months (9).

Intestiphage is a cocktail containing phages targeting 25 different pathogenic enteric bacteria, and is frequently used to deal with diarrhoea and other gastrointestinal infections. The second cocktail, *Pyophage,* is intended for use in purulent infections and contains phages targeting *Staphylococcus aureus*, several species of *Streptococcus, Pseudomonas aeruginosa*, 2 *Proteus* species and *E.coli* (9,23). If these standard cocktail should prove ineffective or if the patient is suffering from a different type of infection, different phages may be added to the treatment. These phages may be taken from the Eliava Institute's extensive collection, or be isolated from environmental sources, using the patient's own bacteria to select them (23). Similar products are also being marketed in Russia, and are reportedly used extensively in many parts of the country (9).

With its current mode of operation of support through collaborative projects, the Eliava Institute remains a highly active and competent player in the scientific arena of phage therapy. This is evident through the development of the new generation of biodegradable polymeric bandage PhagoBioDerm, and its efforts to set the stage for a "bacteriophage-regulations" in the European Union in cohort with the Queen Astrid Military Hospital in Brussels (14).

As described earlier, most of the use and trials conducted in the Soviet Union had not been published in English. However, during the past two decades many of these studies and knowledge have been translated and made accessible. Several comprehensive reviews have been undertaken in the last few years in order to present these pioneering studies (9,11,14,18,23). One can deduce from these reviews that most of the studies and trials conducted in the Soviet Union does not readily meet the Western criteria of scientific quality. That is, the majority of the trials lack control groups, or the authors fail to supply the information needed for rigorous evaluation of their conclusions. Very often, the methods used by the investigators are also poorly described. Thus, one cannot use these studies as definitive proof for neither efficacy nor safety of phage therapy. One can, however, use these studies and trials as circumstantial evidence and strong indicators for the potential of phage therapy, and one can learn much about modes of clinical application, patient response and about phage therapy as a regular part of medical practice (9).

A study notable for its size and use of control group was a study performed in Tbilisi in 1963 and 1964. It involved the use of bacteriophages for prophylaxis against bacterial dysentery, and included 30,769 children, ranging from 6 months to 7 years of age. In this study, a group of 17,044 children received *Shigella* phages orally once a week, while the remaining group of 13,725 children did not. All children were controlled every week, and faecal samples were tested in all children having enteric infections. This trial showed an incidence of clinically confirmed dysentery 3.8 times higher in the control group, than in the phage treated group (11).

Another clinical trial noteworthy for its use of the double-blind format, but also a general deficiency of information with regard to methodology, was performed in 1982-1983 on soldiers of the Red Army. This trial also aimed to investigate the efficacy of bacteriophage for prophylaxis and treatment of bacterial dysentery. All information about patients, their location and treatment was coded, and the authors reported 10-fold higher occurrence of bacterial dysentery in the placebo group than in the phage treated group (11). Unfortunately, it may seem that the Red Army was a bit too clever in coding their information, because information on the number of patients in each groups and the methods used to evaluate the results, was not made available (23).

Much of the efforts at the Eliava Institute and the rest of the USSR was directed towards treating enteric infections as phage therapy caused far less disruption of the physiological gut flora, compared to that of antibiotics (9). Another major area of clinical application was, and still is, the treatment of surgical and wound infections where conventional antibiotics proved inefficient, such as in diabetic foot infections, chronic osteomyelitis and in multidrug resistant infections (23).

One trial involving purulent infections was conducted in 1974: 236 patients with antibiotic-resistant osteomyelitis, lung abscesses, peritonitis, and postsurgical wound infections caused by *Staphylococci, Streptococci,* and *Proteus* were given the aforementioned phage cocktail "Pyophage" subcutaneously and through surgical drains daily for 5-10 days. The investigators reported the complete elimination of pathogenic bacteria in 92 % of the patients (18).

Perhaps the most detailed Soviet time study into bacteriophage therapy was conducted at the Institute of Oncology in Moscow in 1989. In total 131 cancer patients with postsurgical wound infections were included in the study and divided into two groups. While one group of 66 patients served as control group, receiving antibiotics only, the other group (n=65) was subdivided into three subgroups: The first subgroup received bacteriophages and antibiotics concurrently from the onset of suppurative infection. The second subgroup received phage therapy after antibiotic therapy had failed, and the third subgroup received phage therapy only. Three types of phages were employed, depending on the pathogen; anti-staphylococcus, anti-pseudomonas and the pyophage cocktail. The authors reported positive clinical results in 81.5 % of the phage treated patients, compared to 60.6 % in the control group. They were also able to report that the efficacy of the anti-pseudomonas and anti-staphylococcus phages were considerably greater, with 86.7 % and 74.4 % respectively, than for the pyophage cocktail with 57,1 % (18). These results are important because they give further indications and substance to the belief that phage therapy is more effective when using phages selected based on the relevant pathogenic bacteria, as compared to the use of preformed phage cocktails.

The four trials described above were chosen on the basis that they illustrate the research and use of phage therapy in the Soviet Union, in a good manner. Other studies that also merit being mentioned here are included in table 3, having been reviewed and cited by Abedon and Sulakvelidze (9,11). It is also important to note that phage therapy was, and still is, a part of standard medical care in Georgia and Russia (23).

Table 3 - Overview of phage therapy studies in the USSR (9,11).

Publication	Year	Aetiology	Disease	*n,* patients	Comments
Markoishvili *et al.*	2002	*E.coli, Proteus, Pseudomonas, Staphylococcus*	Ulcers and wounds	96	70% success
Lazareva *et al.*	2001	*Proteus, Staphylococcus, Streptococcus*	Burn wounds	54	Pyophage; Reduced septic complications, fever and number of colonizing bacteria
Perepanova *et al.*	1995	*E.coli, Proteus, Staphylococcus*	Acute and chronic urogenital inflammation	46	Adapted phages used; 92 % showed significant clinical improvement, 84 % bacteriological clearance
Miliutina	1993	*Salmonella, Shigella*	Salmonellosis and dysentery	?	Found advantage in the use of phage and antibiotics in combination
Bogovazova *et al.*	1992	*K.ozaenae, K.pneumoniae, K.rhinoscleromatis*	Infections of skin and nasal mucosa	109	Adapted phages used and reported to be effective in treating *Klebsiella* infections in all included patients.
Sakandelidze *et al.*	1991	*E.coli, P.aeruginosa, Proteus, Staphylococcus, Streptococcus, Enterococcus*	Infectious allergoses	1380	360 patients treated with phages, 404 treated with antibiotics and 576 patients treated with combined phages and antibiotics. Clinical improvement observed in 86, 48, and 83 % of the cases, respectively.
Kochetkova *et al.*	1989	*Pseudomonas, Staphylococcus*	Postoperative wound infections in cancer patients	131	82% successful *vs.* 61% in antibiotic control group.
Anpilov, Prokudin	1984	*Shigella*	Dysentery	?	10-fold lower incidence of dysentery in phage-treated group.
Martymova *et al.*	1984	*P.aeruginosa*	Prophylactic	27	Normalization of microflora in infected sites with IgA production stimulated
Meladze *et al.*	1982	*Staphylococcus*	Lung and pleural infections	223	82 % made full recovery with phages *vs* 64 % with antibiotics.
Tolkacheva *et al.*	1981	*E.coli, Proteus, Shigella*	Enteric infections	59	Immunosuppressed leukaemia patients. Better results when given in combination with bifidobacteria.
Isoeliani *et al.*	1980	*E.coli, Proteus, Staphylococcus, Streptococcus*	Lung and pleural infections	45	Successful phage use in combination with antibiotics.
Litvinova *et al.*	1978	*E.coli, Proteus*	Intestinal dysbacteriosis	500	Successful treatment of premature infants.
Zhukov-Verezhnikov *et al.*	1978	*E.coli, Proteus, Staphylococcus, Streptococcus*	Purulent Infections	60	Improved efficacy using phages selected against bacterial strains isolated from individual patients versus commercial phage preparations.
Pipiia *et al.*	1976		Abscessing pneumonia	?	Multiple treatment approaches including use of phages
Sakandelidze *et al.*	1974	*Proteus, Staphylococcus, Streptococcus*	Purulent infections	236	92 % recovered fully.
Babalova *et al.*	1967	*Shigella*	Bacterial dysentery	30,796	Phages used successfully for prophylaxis of bacterial dysentery

Although, many more studies were undertaken and phages were used in the everyday clinical care of patients in the Soviet Union, these studies and experiences were not made available to the international community (14). However, much of these undertakings, efforts and knowledge from the archives of the Eliava Institute have recently been summarized, comprehensively covered and published in an extensive review from Dr. Nina Chanishvili (24).

8.2.6 Poland

The city of Wroclaw, Poland, with a long history dedicated to bacteriophage research and treatment is the seat of another major centre, the Hirszfeld Institute of Immunology and Experimental Therapy, founded in 1952 (ref.(25)). Whereas the Eliava Institute focused its efforts on phage cocktails and enjoyed the fact that phage therapy is a standard part of the Georgian medical system, the Hirszfeld Institute has developed an individualized approach where adapted phages are carefully chosen and employed in cases where antibiotic treatment has failed (23). In order to conduct this method efficiently they have utilized the concept of a "phage bank", where different bacteriophages and phage preparations are stored, ready to be tested for efficacy against bacterial isolates, before they are employed to the patient. The Hirszfeld Institutes bacteriophage collection stems back to 1948 and contains today more than 500 virulent bacteriophages (table 4).

Table 4 - Bacteriophage collection at the Hirszfeld Institute, May 2011, according to Miedzybrodzki (25).

Bacteria	Number of different phages
Escherichia coli	121
Klebsiella pneumoniae or Klebsiella oxytoca	95
Enterococcus faecalis or Enterococcus faecium	73
Enterobacter cloacae	48
Shigella flexneri or Shigella sonnei	39
Citrobacter freundii	38
Pseudomonas aeruginosa or Pseudomonas fluorescens	37
Salmonella enteritidis or Salmonella typhimurium	32
Stenotrophomonas maltophilia	18
Serratia marcescens or Serratia liquefaciens	17
Proteus mirabilis	17
Morganella morganii	14
Staphylococcus aureus	7
Acinetobacter baumannii	5
Burkholderia cepacia	2

The Hirszfeld Institute is the source of the most detailed studies of bacteriophage therapy, that have been published in English language journals (11). In addition to performing clinical trials assessing the efficacy of phage therapy, the Hirszfeld Institute has also published extensively on the interaction between bacteriophages and the human immune system (8,26–28).

Under Polish law, bacteriophage therapy is considered as experimental therapy. This means that all patients have to formally consent to receiving phage therapy, their case must be approved by institutional review board and all other available treatment options must have failed (14,23). This means that the Hirszfeld Institute has a distinctively different mode of operation than the Eliava Institute has. Traditionally, none of the therapeutic efforts have taken place at the Hirszfeld Institute itself, but instead at local clinics and regional hospitals on a case-to-case basis (23). Detailed records of these treatments were kept and their results published, and will to some extend be discussed in the sections below. Since these studies and trials were not blinded and since antibiotics often were used in parallel with phages, they are met with the same type of criticism and scepticism as the earlier described Soviet studies (9,23). However, in 2005, after Poland's integration into the European Union, the Hirszfeld Institute opened its own clinic, the Phage Therapy Unit, dedicated to the treatment of antibiotic-resistant infections. With this new setting in terms of both facilities and EU-regulations, the Hirszfeld Institute is now working towards controlled clinical trials (23).

Below follows a description of the most notable studies undertaken at the Hirszfeld Institute from its beginning until present (table 5). Although many of the studies listed in the table below will not be discussed here, that have been comprehensively review and cited by Sulakvelidze and Alisky (11,18).

As the bacteriophage enthusiasm wave spread over Europe in the 1920s and 1930s, Poland proved to be no exception. With the earliest reported use of phage therapy in 1925, a culture for using adapted phages emerged during the 1940s (23). While the Hirszfeld Institute was established in 1952, publications of results during its first two decades of operation remains scarce. However, in the early 1980s Hirszfeld director Stefan Slopek together with his colleagues, published a series of six articles on the effectiveness of phage therapy against various types of infections (11). Their seventh article summarized the results of all these studies, and merits further discussion (29).

In 1987, Slopek *et al.* report on the bacteriophage treatment of 550 patients with bacterial septicaemia in the years 1981 – 1986. The patients' age ranged from 1 week to 86 years, and they were treated at 10 different hospitals, in three different cities. Antibiotic therapy was reported to be ineffective in 518 of the patients, prior to commencement of phage therapy. The causative organisms were identified as *Staphylococci, Pseudomonas, Escherichia, Klebsiella*, and *Salmonella*. All patients received adapted phages from the Hirszfeld Institute collection, and the phages were administered orally, topically, intra-pleural/peritoneal, as eye drops, or as nose spray. The duration of treatment ranged from one to 16 weeks, with phages being administrated up to 14 days after negative bacterial cultures were acquired. The authors report an overall success rate of 92 % (11,18,29).

This study is notable since it provides evidence of the benefits of phage therapy, especially when one takes into account that in the majority of patients, antibiotic therapy had already failed. There are however, several flaws and drawbacks to this study: Firstly, a control group receiving antibiotics or placebo is not included. Secondly, information on the type of antibiotics used before and in parallel with phages are not provided. Thirdly, the treatment was conducted at several different hospitals under different conditions, and data may not have been reported to the Institute in full detail (23).

In 2000, Weber-Dabrowska summarises phage therapy under the direction of the Hirszfeld Institute in the years 1987 – 1999 (22). In this period, 1307 patients with multidrug resistant suppurative infections were treated with adapted bacteriophages. All patients received 10 ml (children 5 ml) of bacteriophage solutions three times daily before meals and after neutralization of the gastric juice. The patients also received local administration of bacteriophages, depending on the localization of the infectious focus. As in the Slopek paper, and due to the organization of the Hirszfeld Institute at the time, therapy was carried out at several different hospitals and clinics, and lasted 32 days on average. The authors reported full recovery in 85.9 % of the patients, with only 3.8 % having no effect of the phage therapy, with a 100 % cure-rate in purulent meningitis and furunculosis. Moreover, the authors point out that phages were particularly effective in treating staphylococci and pseudomonas, with cure-rates of 95 % and 89 % respectively.

These seemingly very impressive results can be taken as a good indication for the effectiveness of phage therapy, but not much more. As with the Slopek paper, the study by Weber-Dabrowska does not include the necessary information needed for proof of efficacy. Information on concurrent use of antibiotics, procedures for standardization and the lack of control groups, are some of the points missing.

A recent paper from 2012 Ryszard Miedzybrodzki *et al.*, accounts for the progress and treatment of patients at the Phage Therapy Unit at the Hirszfeld Institute in the years 2008 – 2010 (25). Refreshingly, this very comprehensive and detailed report contains in depth information on the current status and the maintenance of the phage bank, the preparation of therapeutic phage lysates, detailed patient inclusion and exclusion criteria, a sound methodology for assessing the efficacy of the treatment, thorough monitoring of side effects and immunological response and a systematic statistical analysis of data. It should be noted that even this study does not include a control group, and is rather a statistical review of a case series than a clinical trial *per se*.

Miedzybrodzki reports on the treatment of 153 patients treated at the Phage Therapy Unit for a wide assortment of multidrug resistant and treatment resistant infections, using adapted phages. Dosing, administration and monitoring of the patients status were standardized according to the Institutes treatment protocol. Good clinical improvement was seen in 40 % of the patients, with complete recovery or pathogen eradication proven by two consecutive negative bacterial cultures in 20 %. These rates of efficacy are significantly lower than the results previously published by the Hirszfeld Institute or the Eliava Institute, however much more detailed, credible, and well supported.

These considerably lower positive results, may be because in contrast to earlier studies all patients were treated under the direct control and supervision of the Institute, and assessed against a strict monitoring protocol. The authors point out, that by this method and evaluation they were able to achieve complete recovery in one out of every five patients that were resistant to antibiotic therapy, and more importantly, through their thorough monitoring of laboratory parameters and side effects they were able to provide substantial documentation supporting the belief that phage therapy is safe.

The studies and case reports originating from the Hirszfeld Institute from before 2005 have obvious scientific limitations. They are however important in that they provide invaluable expertise and knowledge of the clinical application of phage therapy and of its safety. However, one can observe a clear shift in the mode of operation and scientific approach after the opening of the Phage Therapy Unit. The new studies deriving from the Institutes own clinic are clearly adapted to EU regulations and have taken a huge step towards providing the type of quality phage research that have been missing.

Table 5 - Overview of phage therapy in Poland, reviewed by Sulakvelidze and Alisky (11,18).

Publication	Year	Aetiology	Disease	n, patients	Comments
Miedzybrodzki et al.(25)	2012	Diverse	Chronic, treatment resistant infections	153	Patients at PTU 2008-2010. 40 % Good clinical response, 20 % with complete pathogen eradication. Refined methods. See discussion in the text.
Weber-Dabrowska et al.(28)	2006	Staphylococcus homis, Staphylococcus epidermidis	Otitis media	1	24-year old woman with treatment resistant post-influenza otitis media, successfully treated with phages in combination with lactoferrin.
Weber-Dabrowska et al.(22)	2000	Proteus, S.aureus, E.coli, Klebsiella, Pseudomonas, Enterobacter	Multidrug resistant infections	1307	Patients treated at different hospitals with phage supplied by the Hirszfeld Institute, 1987-1999. Full recovery reported in 85.9%. See discussion in the text.
Stroj et al.	1999	K. pneumoniae	Cerebrospinal meningitis	1	Orally administered phages were used successfully to treat meningitis in a new-born.
Kwarcinski et al.	1994	E.coli	Recurrent subphrenic abscess	1	Recurrent subphrenic abscess after stomach resection, successfully treated.
Cislo et al.	1987	Pseudomonas, Staphylococcus, Klebsiella, Proteus, E.coli	Suppurative skin infections	31	74 % success rate in treating chronically infected skin ulcer with phages orally and locally.
Kucharewicz-Krukowska and Slopek	1987	Pseudomonas, Staphylococcus, Klebsiella, Proteus, E.coli	Various infections	57	Immunogenicity of therapeutic phages was analysed, and the authors concluded that the phages immunogenicity did not inhibit therapy.
Slopek et al.(29)	1987	Pseudomonas, Staphylococcus, Klebsiella, Salmonella, E.coli	Bacterial septicaemia	550	92 % success rate, see discussion in the text.
Weber-Dabrowska et al.	1987	Staphylococcus and gram negative bacteria	Suppurative infections	56	Study to assess the bioavailability of phages after oral administration. Phages found to reach blood and urine.

8.2.7 France

Most available literature on phage therapy and bacteriophage history focuses on the efforts in Poland and the Soviet Union after the collapse of mainstream phage interest in Western Europe and North America. From reviews, one can easily develop the impression that phage therapy disappeared completely in these areas. Although scarcely described in modern literature reviews there was active use of and research into phage therapy in France up until the 1990s (9). The continued use and research was mostly published in French, a language barrier that may have led to this work to be ignored by other authors.

Only in 2011, Stephen T. Abedon and colleagues, published an extensive review on bacteriophage therapy where they place great emphasis on the French experience, after having translated the original French works themselves (9).

The continued use of phage therapy in France was supported by the fact that the Pasteur Institute through the Pasteur Bacteriophage Service continued to produce phage cocktails until the mid-1990s, with the commercial phages originally developed by Felix d'Hérelle being available until 1978. Similarly, detailed reports on the use of phage therapy continued to be published up until 1979. Table 6 gives a brief overview of notable French papers, which are discussed in detail in reference 9.

Table 6 - Overview of phage therapy research in France, according to Abedon et al., (9).

Publication	Year	Aetiology	Disease	n, patients	Comments
Lang et al.	1979	Proteus, Klebsiella, Staphylococcus, Enterobacter, Providencia	Chronic orthopaedic infections	7	Five of the patients successfully treated, though after the removal of implants.
Vieu	1975			n.a.	A review summarizing the phage collection and phage-requests at the Pasteur Bacteriophage Service.
Vieu	1961			n.a.	A review from the Pasteur Bacteriophage Service. Summarizes the knowledge and use of phage therapy in France at the time (9).
Mikeladze	1936	Salmonella typhi	Typhoid fever	21	21 patients treated with phages, compared to 64 patients receiving standard care. Mortality rate reduced from 15.6 % to 4.8 %.
Tsouloukidze	1936	Salmonella typhi	Typhoid fever with intestinal perforation	?	Administration of phages into the peritoneal cavity during surgical laparotomy. Reduced mortality from 85 % to 20 %.
Gougerot, Peyre	1936	Various	Skin infections, recurrent furnuculosis.	?	Patients treated with local administration of phages. Reportedly good results.
Sauve	1936	Staphylococcus	Septicaemia	9	Report of successful intravenous phage treatment of 9 patients with septicaemia.
Michon	1936	Various	Urinary tract infections	?	Reportedly muss less relapse with phage treatment compared to silver nitrate treatment.

As shown above, active work on phage therapy in humans was more or less absent in most of Western Europe and North America. However, scientists started to use bacteriophages as a genetic tool, opening a whole new field of science (19). Thus, research on bacteriophages continued outside the Soviet Union, Poland, and France, although not with the focus on using phages to treat human infections.

8.2.8 Renewed Interest in Phage Therapy

The 1982 paper of Smith and Higgins is often accredited for revitalizing the interest in phage therapy (9,18,19). They described the use of phage to treat *E.coli* infections in mice, which spawned more research in the years to come, especially in animal models (18).

During the late 1990s, belief that bacteriophages could be developed as drugs according to western guidelines were strong and several private companies joined the race. At the turn of the millennia, several of these companies were preparing to undertake double blind, randomized, placebo controlled clinical trials. However, due to the stock-market crisis in 2001, funding for these trials was obviously lost (23).

These companies and others switched their efforts into developing phage products for use into agricultural, animal and food use, with some products already having reached approval from the American Food and Drug Administration (FDA) (30). This success in developing and gaining approval for phage products has once again rejuvenated the drive towards developing therapeutic phages for human use. This has resulted in several recent small clinical trials, which will be presented in detail below.

8.2.8.1 Nestlé Safety Trial

In 2005, researchers at the Nestlé Research Center in Lausanne, Switzerland, described a phage therapy safety test, performed on healthy volunteers, using the *E.coli* T4 bacteriophage (31). The study was designed as a randomized, double-blinded, placebo-controlled study with three-period crossover. Fifteen healthy adult volunteers received either a high dose of phages (10^5 PFU/ml) in their drinking water, a lower dose (10^3 PFU/ml), or placebo. The preparations were administered orally 3 times a day for two consecutive days, followed by a five-day monitoring period. Over the four week trial period, where the first week served as a baseline control, all volunteers thus received all three preparations, and a comparison was made.

All volunteers underwent clinical examination at day 0 and day 30, where blood samples were taken and analysed. In addition, stool samples were taken two times during the first week, and every day during the last three weeks of the trial. The authors reported only five cases of mild adverse events not warranting treatment, such as increased peristalsis and nausea. The events were unrelated to the dose of phage ingested. Moreover, for all volunteers; liver functions tests remained normal, no T4 phages were detectable in serum, and T4-specific antibodies were not observed. Additionally, faecal phage counts correlated in a dose-dependent manner with the orally applied dose.

The T4 phage has been chosen for this trial because it is one of the best described and characterised phages. Furthermore, it does not contains known virulence genes, making it suitable for such a trial, but not for future use as a therapeutic phage. The authors showed that 7.1 % of the *E.coli* colonies in the volunteers were susceptible to the T4 phage before the trial, compared to only 0.9% after. Thus, the authors conclude that the treatments were well tolerated and safe, and more importantly provided a good example of a scientifically sound human phage therapy study.

The same authors participated in a similar trial conducted in Bangladesh, which was published in 2012 (32). This study followed the same study design as in the 2005 safety trial, but used a well-described 9-phage cocktail instead of the mono-phage preparation. Again, no serious adverse reactions were reported.

8.2.8.2   Biocontrol Phase I/II Trial on Chronic Otitis Externa

In 2009, the British company Biocontrol Ltd., undertook a phase I/II clinical trial on patients with antibiotic-resistant *Pseudomonas aeruginosa* chronic otitis (33). The trial was conducted in collaboration with the University College London Ear Institute and Royal National Throat, Nose and Ear Hospital in London.

Earlier on, Biocontrol Ltd., had reported the successful use of a bacteriophage cocktail for antibiotic-resistant *Pseudomonas aeruginosa* chronic otitis in dogs (34). The same phage cocktail, Biophage-PA, a cocktail that contains six phages sensitive to different strains of *P. aeruginosa*, was used in 2009.

The 2009 trial was designed as a randomised, double blind, placebo-controlled phase I/II clinical trial. In all, 24 patients were included in the study, and randomized into two groups of twelve treated with either a single dose of Biophage-PA or placebo and followed up at 7, 21 and 42 days after treatment by the same otolaryngologist.

The main outcome measurements were physician assessed clinical condition, and patient assessed condition, both using a Visual Analogue Scale (VAS). Bacterial and phage counts were also conducted initially and at follow up examinations.

The authors reported significant clinical improvement and reductions in bacterial counts in the phage treated group, with no treatment related adverse events observed. All patients in the treated group improved, with a mean VAS reduction of 50 %. Interestingly, in three of the twelve phage treated patients (25 % of the patients), a complete eradication and full recovery was achieved.

Of note, the authors also point to the finding that the mean duration of active bacteriophage replication and proliferation in the test group was 23 days, arguing that one should consider repeating treatment every three weeks. Based on these positive results, the undertakers of this trial are now preparing a larger, multicentre, phase III, clinical trial. However, this 2009 study remains to date the only phase I/II clinical trial on phage therapy in human infections that come close to the gold standard on how clinical trials on bacteriophage therapeutics should be conducted (35).

8.2.8.3 Belgian Trial on Burn Patients

In 2009, Researchers at the Queen Astrid Military Hospital in Brussels, Belgium, published details on the production and quality control of a three-phage cocktail, targeting *P. aeruginosa* and *S.aureus*, and its administration to a small cohort of burn patients (20). The Burn Wound Centre at the Queen Astrid Military Hospital undertook this study as a small clinical safety trial, as a pretext for a full worthy clinical trial using bacteriophages to treat infected burn wounds (36).

The authors style in detail the production and purification techniques used, and the quality control of stability, pyrogenicity, sterility, cytotoxicity, and confirmation of the absence of temperate phages. Complete genome-analyses were performed in order to rule out the presence of any toxin-coding genes.

Moreover, the safety trial also included the testing of the phage cocktail on burn patients. The cocktail was administered as a spray on one part of the wound, while a distant part served as control receiving standard therapy. Both regions were monitored with tissue biopsies, and the patients were carefully monitored for three weeks following the treatment (23).

While no adverse events were reported, the details of the effect on patients are not yet published. However, this study is notable and important for its wide-ranging and careful description and methodology in the production of a therapeutic phage cocktail. In this respect, the study meets the criteria and benchmark in phage therapy clinical trials as described by Helena Parracho in 2012 (ref.(35)).

8.2.8.4 Texas Safety Trial

The results of a physician-initiated, FDA-approved, phase I, prospective, randomized, double-blind clinical trial, conducted at the Wound Care Center in Lubbock, Texas, were published in 2009 (26). The study was designed to evaluate the safety of the bacteriophage cocktail "WPP-201", prepared by Alexander Sulakvelidze at Intralytix. The cocktail contained eight different phages; five for *P.aeruginosa*, two for *S.aureus* and one for *E.coli*. All eight phages chosen for this cocktail were thoroughly characterized by means of genome sequencing, protein fingerprint profile, plaque morphology, and taxonomy. This extensive preparatory work, carried out by Intralytix, was essential for getting FDA approval for the trial (23).

The patients included in the trial all had full thickness venous leg ulcers of more than 30 days´ duration, with or without clinical signs of infection. In all, 42 patients were included in the trial, of which 39 completed the treatment, 18 in the treatment group and 21 in the control. The phage preparation or placebo was applied through sonication, using an ultrasound device, once a week for the duration of twelve weeks. In addition, all patients received the same care in terms of wound management, which included special dressings and a topical gel containing lactoferrin and xylitol.

The authors reported no significant adverse effects of the phage therapy, and concluded that the "WPP-201" bacteriophage cocktail did not raise any safety concerns with regard to human use. However, not a part of the primary endpoint or study design, the efficacy of the phage cocktail was nonetheless analysed. This analysis revealed no noteworthy differences between the control and treatment groups. Kutter *et al.* attributed the apparent lack of efficacy of the bacteriophage cocktail to the fact that the wound bacterial flora was not tested for sensitivity to the phage cocktail prior to the trial. Furthermore, they argue that the parallel use of lactoferrin and application through sonication can contributed to bacteriophage interference and inactivation.

In all, in the century that have passed since the discovery of bacteriophages, they have been praised as a miracle cure, condemned as a flop, forgotten and rediscovered in the West. In the meantime, phage therapy gained foothold as a standard treatment in the Soviet Union, an experience we can learn much from today.

8.3   Virology of Bacteriophages

Bacteriophages make up a diverse group of viruses that share the common trait of infecting bacteria and archaea. Virtually omnipresent in nature, they play a vital role in effectively every ecosystem. It is estimated that a total of 1×10^{30} to 1×10^{32} phage particles exist at any one time, giving approximately 10 bacteriophages to every single bacterium (10,12). The activity of bacteriophages is responsible for killing an expected one-half of the bacterial population worldwide every 48 hours. This co-existence between bacteria and bacteriophages has lasted for billions of years, with bacteria constantly trying to avoid the phages by altering their appearance and mechanisms through mutations, and phages responding in kind to adapt at an even more rapid rate (37).

These "eaters of bacteria" are packed full of information and potential, and have been the subject of much research. In the chapters below, the details of their biology will be briefly explored.

8.3.1   Classification

Bacteriophages constitute a diverse group of viruses. They are divided into 13 families and 30 genera (table 7). Since 1959 over 6000 different bacteriophages have been identified by electron microscopy, and allocated to their correct family and genus. However, estimates using metagenomics predicts the existence of several 100,000 or even millions of different bacteriophages, which in any case represents the largest viral group in nature (38,39).

Table 7 - Classification of bacteriophages, acc. to International Committee on Taxonomy of Viruses (38,39).

Order	Family	Nucleic acid	Note	n, species
Caudovirales	Myoviridae	dsDNA (L)	T4-phage	1300+
	Siphoviridae	dsDNA (L)	λ-phage	3200+
	Podoviridae	dsDNA (L)	T7-phage	770+
Unassigned	Corticoviridae	dsDNA (C)		3
	Cystoviridae	dsRNA (L,S)		3
	Inoviridae	ssDNA (C)		66
	Leviviridae	ssRNA (L)		38
	Microviridae	ssDNA (C)		38
	Plasmaviridae	dsDNA (C)		5
	Tectiviridae	dsDNA (L)	Infects both bacteria and archaea	19
	Fuselloviridae	dsDNA (C)	Infects archaea	8
Ligamenvirales	Rudiviridae	dsDNA (L)	Infects archaea	2
	Lipothrixviridae	dsDNA (L)	Infects archaea	6

Table 8 - Footnote to table 7.

Abbreviation	Meaning
ds	Double-stranded
ss	Single-stranded
L	Linear
C	Circular
S	Segmented

8.3.2   Structure, and basic properties

Being a highly diverse group of viruses, they display a variety of different structural elements, shapes, and properties (Fig. 5). The common trait is that they all contain a core of nucleic acid, contained within a protein or lipoprotein capsid (12). The range in morphology, nucleic acid and other elements such as an envelope, gives an enormous variety to the group. Therefore, a more detailed description and study of all these elements lies outside the scope of this review. However, a descriptive presentation of the representative order Caudovirales follows below.

The order Caudovirales, representing the families Myoviridae, Siphoviridae and Podoviridae, and hence over 96% of all phages, is characterised by its icosahedral head, a neck and a tail with special fibres used for attachment to target bacteria (Fig. 6). The viruses in this order all contain dsDNA (L), contained within a protein capsid. As the length and sequence of the genomes varies greatly within each family and genus, ranging from 17,000 to 700,000 base pairs, they are classified together based on their distinctive morphology. Also called tailed bacteriophages, with tail lengths between 10 to 800 nm, their tail can be contractile as in the *Myoviridae* family, long and noncontractile as in the *Siphoviridae* family, or short and noncontractile as in the *Podoviridae* family (39).

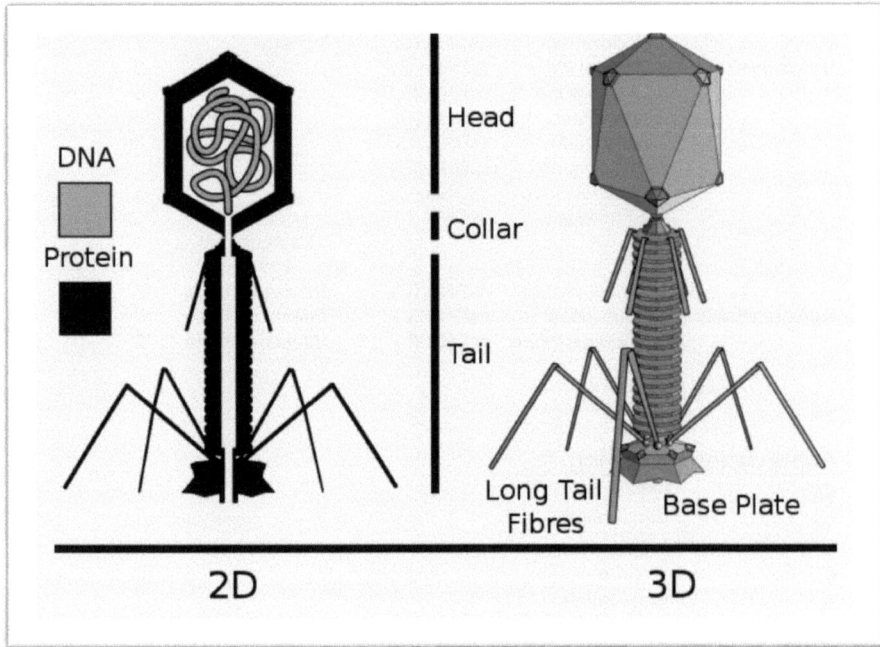

Figure 5 - Schematic drawing of Myoviridae. Source: Wikimedia Commons

8.3.3 Mechanism of Action and Life Cycle

As stated earlier, bacteriophages exhibit specificity in terms of which bacteria they are able to infect. A phage is usually specific for a bacterial species or several strains of the same species. Polyvalent phages that have a host range across species or genera, are few in number (12,40). The more than 6,000 bacteriophages that have been classified and studied to date, are able to infect at least 130 bacterial genera (39).

All bacteriophages express fibres through which they can interact with bacterial surface receptors. For the phages belonging to the order *Caudovirales,* these fibres extend from the tail, while non-tailed phages express tooth-like fibres from their capsid or head. However, since phages are immotile, they depend on chance encounters with the right receptors. If the phage is specific for the bacterium, an irreversible attachment, an adsorption, to the surface receptors occurs (12,39,41,42).

Once, an irreversible attachment is made, the phage will penetrate the bacterial cell wall and membrane, and inject its genetic material into the bacterium (Fig. 7). *Myoviridae* family phages use their hollow, contractile tail as a syringe to gain entry to the bacteria, while the phages with a noncontractile tail and non-tailed phages employ the use of enzymes to degrade a portion of the cell wall, before inserting their genome (37,41).

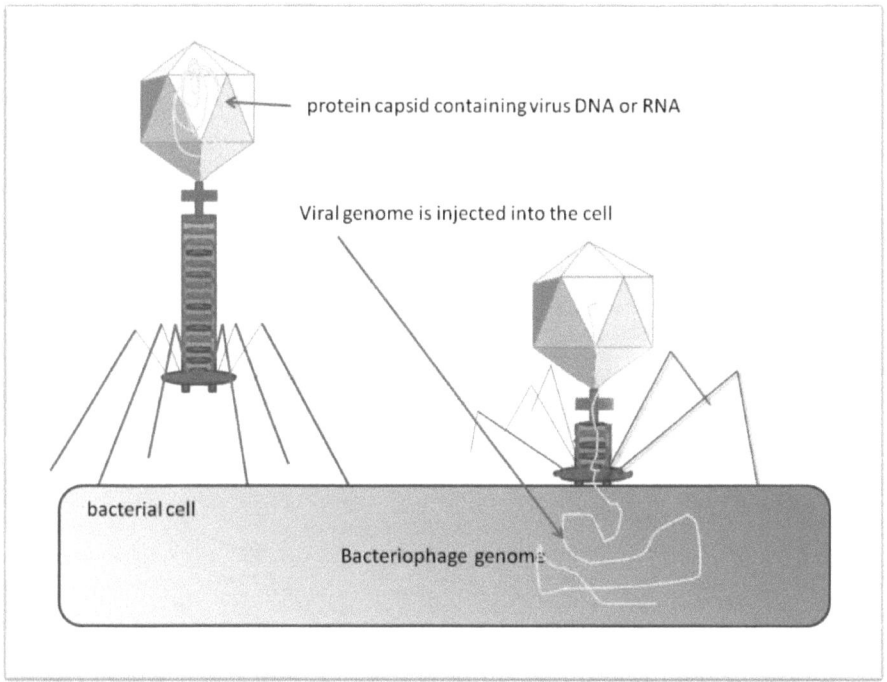

Figure 6 - Myoviridae injection. Source: Wikimedia Commons

Once the phage genome has been introduced to the bacteria, the phage may follow either the lysogenic or lytic life cycle (Fig. 8) (ref.(12)). Phages that follows the lysogenic life cycle are called temperate phages as they simply integrate their genome into the host genome. There it remains inactive as a prophage, only replicating together with the host. The prophage may later become active and enter a lytic life cycle if the bacteria encounters adverse environments or otherwise mobilises it (42).

[37]

Phages that follow the lytic cycle are called virulent phages and are chosen for traditional phage therapy. After injection of the phage genome into the host, viral mRNA will be translated into proteins by the bacterial ribosomes. These proteins play a vital role in hijacking the bacterial machinery and start replication of the phage genome, and synthesis of structural proteins that are required for the assembly of new phages. As the phage genome is replicated, normal bacterial synthetic and metabolic processes are shut down, and the newly replicated phage genome is assembled into new phage virions. In all, 100 – 300 new virions are rapidly produced and then released into its surroundings, when lysis of the bacterium occurs. Lysis is usually accomplished through the membrane-disturbing effect of the phage coded enzymes holin and endolysin. These new viral progeny are then able to meet new bacteria and repeat the process (12,37,40,42).

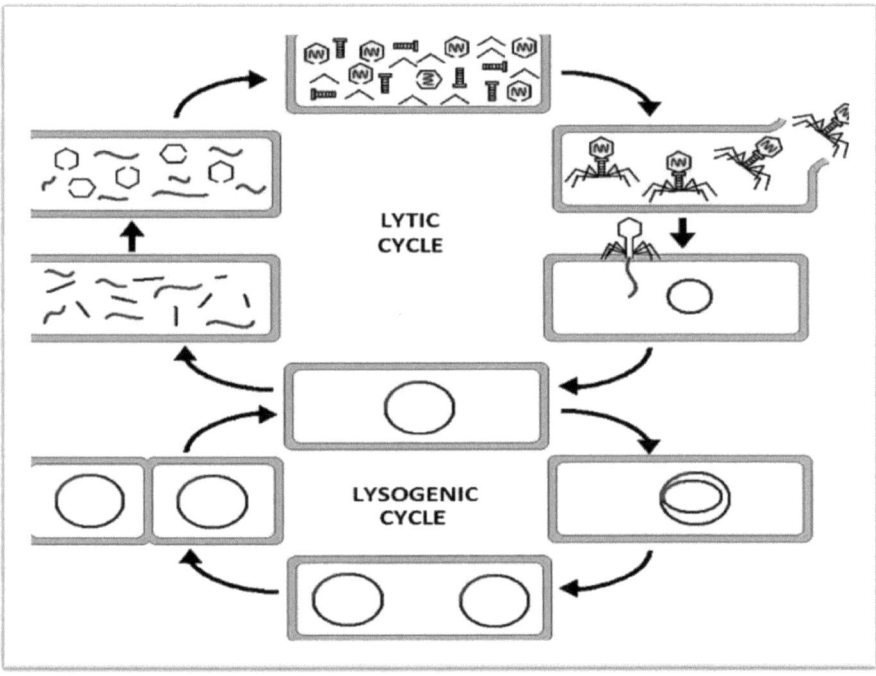

Figure 7 - Lytic and lysogenic life cycle. Source: Wikimedia Commons

8.4   Clinical Application of Bacteriophages

The first and foremost area of application of bacteriophages in clinical medicine are bacterial infections. In the following sections the indications, preparation, and administration of phage

[38]

therapy will be explored. In addition, the employment of bacteriophages in treatment of non-infectious diseases and in diagnostic procedures will also be briefly outlined.

8.4.1 Indications

As earlier mentioned, phage therapy was first used to treat dysentery (23). Diarrheal infections also remained one of the primary areas of focus for the Eliava Institute, which conducted several trials on the topic. As phage therapy evolved into a standard part of the Soviet and later Georgian health care systems, the indications for receiving phage therapy, included all types of bacterial infections (14). The Hirszfeld Institute took a different path where phage therapy was considered experimental and only indicated in antibiotic resistant and/or chronic infections (23).

With the prospect of reintroducing phage therapy in Europe and North-America, it is envisioned that the main indications for phage therapy will be; antibiotic resistant infections, hard-to-treat-infections (such as osteomyelitis, diabetic ulcers and biofilm-forming infections), and finally treatment in patients where antibiotics are counter-indicated (9).

While the above-mentioned indications are very unspecific concerning aetiology, they are useful in demonstrating the areas of clinical infectology where phage therapy may be most useful. Other authors have also proposed sets of indications to phage therapy such as topical use in wound infections, or *P.aeruginosa* infections in patients with cystic fibrosis (7). Even the use of phages to treat outbreaks of multidrug resistant plague and as a measure in controlling outbreaks following bioterrorism has been discussed (23,43,44).

8.4.2 Preparation of Therapeutic Phages

In deciding to initiate phage therapy, there are two major treatment configurations to choose from; preformed phage cocktails or adapted phages. Although a vast variety of methods have been employed to synthesize phage preparations, often with poor results, only the current methods will be described in this section. Needless to say, the first step of any phage therapy should be to identify the causative bacterial agents, preferably by culture or DNA-based sequencing techniques as PCR and microarrays (45,46).

The use of phage cocktails was pioneered by Felix d'Hérelle and his contemporaries, and further developed and used extensively at the Eliava Institute. These phage cocktails may include several phages that are sensitive to widely different bacteria, such as the *"Pyophage"* and *"Intestiphage"* cocktails, or they may include phages that are sensitive to different strains of one species. The idea of preformed phage cocktails is to add several phages that are sensitive to the most common pathogenic bacterial strains, thus giving a broad spectrum. Even though these preformed cocktails can be employed rapidly, even as prophylactic and empirical treatment, they are not necessarily lytic for the patient's disease causing bacteria (9,14,23).

The concept of using adapted phages is that the phages are proven as lytic for the identified bacteria by testing before administration to the patient. It should be noted that often several different phages are employed at once, in order to reduce the possibility of phage resistance, hence giving an adapted phage cocktail. Using adapted phage cocktails have several therapeutic advantages over preformed phage cocktails, as they are more specific and custom made for the individual patient. The administration of several adapted phages as a cocktail is proven to be more efficient than both preformed phage cocktails and the use of a single adapted phage (11,47).

The major difference between preformed and adapted phage cocktails are thus the choice of included phages and time of production. Regardless of this, the production of therapeutic phages includes many steps, which will briefly be described below. A detailed description of the isolation and characterisation of bacteriophages falls outside the scope of this thesis and will not be included here (41).

- Step 1: Phage choice:
    When composing a preformed phage cocktail, phages are chosen based on the prevailing bacterial strains in society, making it an exercise in microbiological public health. The selection of phages for adapted therapy begins with the isolation and identification of the causative bacterial agents, through standard laboratory methods such as cultivation and polymerase chain reaction. The identified bacteria are then tested against bacteriophages in a similar manner as antibiotic sensitivity testing. Phages showing lytic activity against the bacteria are then chosen (20). Ideally, the bacteriophages should beforehand be well characterised by genome sequencing, proven lytic and free from toxin-coding genes (35).

- Step 2: Phage amplification:
    Once the desired phages have been selected, an amplification process is needed. The phage is introduced to a growth medium, on which the identified bacterium is cultivated, where it is allowed to infect and replicate. The phage culture is monitored by factors such as pO_2, pH or time, based on known phage life cycle parameters (47).

- Step 3: Phage purification:

When the phage culture has produced its desired yield, as determined by culture monitoring, the bacteriophages are harvested. This crude lysate may contain endotoxins, bacterial metabolites, nucleic acids, and even live bacteria. Although several methods for purification, both mechanical and chemical, exists, the most recent method of purification includes centrifugation, membrane filtration and toxin removal by endotoxin-ligand affinity chromatography (20,47).

According to the preferred method of administration to the patient, the purified bacteriophages may be used as the active ingredients in either creams, tablets or solutions, they may also be nebulized or used to impregnate special dressings (20,24,47–49). Furthermore, Nina Chanishvili describes in her 2009 review the production of bacteriophages on an industrial scale (24).

Many authors describe the concept of using a phage bank in order to more effectively produce required phage cocktails (45,47,50,51). Whereas institutions such as the Eliava Institute and Hirszfeld Institute maintain their own collections of phages, the concept of a phage bank widens this idea to include stocks of well-characterised, amplified, and ready to use bacteriophages. This would shorten the time from identification of the pathogen until adapted treatment. Amplified stocks of bacteriophages can freeze-dried and stored for up to 20 years, or stored as a lysate at +2 to +5°C for up to one year (45).

8.4.3   Administration to Patient

Phage therapy can be administered to a patient in several different ways, depending on the site of infection. These methods include parenteral, oral, topical, and inhalational administration. In their 2011 review, Ryan *et al.* assessed the efficacy of different routes of administration in claves, chickens, mice, and humans, and concluded that the parenteral route, especially intraperitoneal injection, was the most efficient (52). Moreover, the authors noted that both oral and topical administration also achieved good results, and that phage coating on indwelling medical devices was efficient in hindering biofilm formation.

Dabrowska *et al.* also evaluated the efficacy of different routes of administration, however with the focus on the bacteriophages ability to penetrate and disseminate throughout the body (53). They showed that bacteriophages were able to permeate into the bloodstream after being applied either topically, orally, intramuscularly, intraperitoneally, or intranasally. This shows that one can treat systemic infections by local application. Additionally, they also showed that bacteriophages are able to cross the blood-brain-barrier. However, Bruttin *et al.* refers to findings indicating that the Kupfer cells in the liver phagocytised 99% of all T4-phages within 30 minutes after intravenous injection (31).

Keeping this and key aspects of phage biology in mind when choosing the method of administration, one can easily deduce that a route ensuring contact between phages and pathogenic bacteria should be chosen. In, for example, diabetic ulcers where blood supply to the wound is usually poor, topical treatment in form of a phage-gel or impregnated dressings should be employed. Also, when the infections are localized and limited, such as an abscess, efforts should be made to treat the focus through injections into the abscess, dressings and phage-lavage of the abscess cavity (9).

The Phage Therapy Unit in Wroclaw has been the leading institution in documenting and publishing, in English, their use and application of bacteriophages. The patients received adapted phages orally, topically, intrarectally, intravaginally or as aerosol inhalation. Depending on the site and type of infection, a combination of topical and oral or topical and intrarectal routes of administration was applied. Intrarectal administration provides a good option with respect to systemic infections, since phages absorbed there partially bypass the portal circulation and thus are able to stay in the bloodstream longer. The issue of systemic phage clearance will be further discussed in the chapters covering pharmacology and safety concerns and immunological response.

The patients at the Phage Therapy Unit were treated with phage preparations in the following manner: Topical phage preparations were administered twice daily by irrigation of wounds and fistulae, moist and phage-impregnated dressings, application of nose and eardrops, vaginal irrigation and inhalations. Phages applied through the oral route were given as a liquid solution three times daily, 30 minutes before meals and after neutralisation of gastric juice by sodium carbonate. Phage preparations applied by the intrarectal route were given twice daily, also in the form of liquid solution. All phage preparations given had a phage titre between 10^6 and 10^9 plaque-forming units / ml.

The Phage Therapy Unit is utilising the principle of repeated administrations, thereby not relying only on phage replication *in vivo*, in a similar manner to passive phage therapy. This is in contrast to many other studies, most notably the 2009 clinical trial on chronic otitis in London that utilises the principle of active phage therapy, where only one dose is administered and phage replication *in vivo* is relied upon (33). The principles of active and passive phage therapy will be discussed in detail in the chapter covering bacteriophage pharmacology.

The use of other medications, especially antibiotics, in parallel to phage therapy, is problematic with respect to measurement of efficacy and outcomes. In certain cases it will not be ethically sound to deprive a patient from antibiotics, at least not as long as phage therapy is considered an experimental therapy, a fact that creates several challenges when designing proper clinical trials.

[42]

Monitoring of patients receiving phage therapy depends of course on the clinical condition of the patient. As patients with severe life threatening infections require monitoring at an intensive care unit, others require just an outpatient setting. With regard to monitoring the safety and efficacy of phage therapy, several parameters have been used. Frequent blood tests, including full blood count, liver and kidney function tests, inflammation markers and immunoglobulins have been used to assess the patient's general condition, the immunological response and safety of treatment (25,27).

Measurement of outcome is dependent on the study design and is regrettably not standardized. In the retrospective analysis of the patient's at the Phage Therapy Unit, the results of treatment were evaluated by the physician responsible for the phage therapy and based upon at least two consecutive bacterial cell cultures, assessment of symptoms and inflammation markers (25). In the 2009 chronic otitis trial in London, efficacy was, as previously described, evaluated using a visual analogue scale and bacterial and phage counts (33). This difference in methodology makes it hard to provide an accurate comparison between the two results.

8.4.4   Other Clinical Use of Phages

Bacteriophages have also gained a large role in laboratory practice, where they have been used as tools in molecular biology, especially through the technique called phage display. Phage display is the method where by introducing DNA sequences encoding for proteins of interest into the phage genome, one causes the phage to express this protein and display it. This technique has proven a useful tool in the study of gene-protein interaction and protein engineering, and has laid the groundwork for other methods of bacteriophage application in clinical medicine (41,44,54).

One hypostatised application of bacteriophage is in cancer therapy. As early as in 1940 it was shown that bacteriophages accumulate in and inhibit the growth of tumour tissue, and later, in 1958, it was discovered that bacteriophages are able to bind cancer cells and lymphocytes *in vivo* (53). Also, Gorski *et al.* presented the finding that bacteriophages expressing the KDG+ sequence are able to bind to β3 integrins, which are expressed by platelets, monocytes, some lymphocytes and some neoplastic cells (8). KDG+ phages are by binding the β3 integrin then able to downregulate the activity of these cells.

These findings provide a potential novel method for selectively modifying the behaviour of certain cells, including the prospect of using engineered phages in the treatment of cancer in addition to cardiovascular and autoimmune diseases. In his 2010 review on the rational design of phage therapeutics, Goodridge elaborates on the biotechnological techniques that can be used to modify bacteriophages to express a more desired behaviour (48). By using simple, known, and available methods one can effectively change the host-range of bacteriophages, introduce new genes that code for a non-toxic death of the target cell, and couple phages with other molecules such as chemotherapeutics for enhanced lytic activity or polyethylene glycol to reduce immune system clearance.

Among the techniques described by Goodridge is the modification of a bacteriophage into an engineered viral vector, which is a delivery vehicle for lethal or protective genes. Westwater *et al.* account for the production and application of a viral vector, based on a lysogenic phage to deliver lethal genes into a mouse with bacteraemia (55). Successful in reducing the number of bacteria, the authors conclude that DNA transfer from the phage to the mouse was efficient and asserted the potential for the use of temperate phages as vectors for antimicrobial therapy and as DNA vaccines.

By taking advantage of the nature of bacteriophages and modern knowledge in biotechnology, there are endless opportunities to utilise phages as target-selective drugs, either as a carrier of other therapeutic compounds or as viral vectors. In this way, bacteriophages or products derived from bacteriophages have the prospect to be used in the modification and treatment of a wide range of pathophysiological processes and illnesses. This pathway is already being explored by several private companies and research institutions, as it offers a possible solution to some of the regulatory issues that surround phage therapy (56).

One phage-derived product that shows great promise in *in vivo* animal studies is the use of phage lysins to treat bacterial infections. Lysins are cell hydrolases, enzymes produced by bacteriophages that are able to break down the bacterial cell wall. On the basis of positive outcome in animal studies, the fact that no adverse immunological response was observed and the ease of which one can synthetically mass produce phage lysins, makes it one of the most interesting prospects on the horizon (30). Also, as lysins are enzymes and not viruses they face a wholly different outlook with regard to regulatory approval and intellectual property protection (56).

8.5   Bacteriophage Pharmacology

Compared to the rather large number of papers published on phage therapy since its inception, few actually tackle the issue of phage therapy pharmacology (see appendix for statistics on studies included in this thesis). However, in the last 10-15 years the topic has been brought to the surface by a handful of reviews and original research articles (51,57–60). Because bacteriophages have the potential to be self-amplifying pharmaceuticals, their pharmacological properties must be addressed in a slightly different manner than for conventional antibiotics. In the following sections, the basic pharmacologic principles of phage therapy will be addressed.

8.5.1   Pharmacokinetics of Phage Therapy

The topic of phage pharmacokinetics has received considerably more attention in the literature than its counterpart pharmacodynamics, perhaps due to the peculiar nature of phage pharmacodynamics and the necessity of a well described pharmacokinetic for regulatory approval (51). The subject of pharmacokinetics is the study of the fate of drugs in the human body and concerns the classical constellation of absorption, distribution, metabolism and excretion (61).

Absorption of bacteriophages into the systemic blood circulation follows a variety of administration routes, as previously described (53). Measurements of phage density in blood reveal that phages can move with ease from for example the peritoneal cavity, intestine, anal canal, or muscle into the bloodstream. There is, however, a general lack of studies into the mechanism behind this compartment transfer.

Distribution of bacteriophages in the body, which is from tissue to blood, blood to tissue or tissue to tissue, follows the concentration gradient, and can be easily calculated using standard first-order reaction kinetics. Utilising this principle one can realise that the more phages that are provided at any one place (for example the intestinal lumen), the greater the forward movement of phage (into the bloodstream) will be (51).

Metabolism of bacteriophages is analogous to the population kinetics of bacteriophages, and is at least a two-fold concept to examine as it concerns phage replication and phage decay. Through their natural life cycle virulent bacteriophages replicate greatly in number, where any one phage is able to produce up to 300 progeny (10). This self-amplification allows one to consider several dosing options, as will be discussed below. Phage decay, although a part of the removal process of bacteriophages, is also a metabolic matter. Phage decay can occur as a consequence of inactivation by restriction endonucleases present in bacteria, or through structural damage caused by unfavourable pH values and protein denaturing enzymes e.g. in the intestinal lumen (51).

Removal of bacteriophages from the bloodstream is effectively done by the reticuloendothelial system. As previously cited, a study found that 99% of all phages were phagocytised within 30 minutes following intravenous injection. The bacteriophages are recognised by the reticuloendothelial system based on protein motifs that they are displaying. Using this to an advantage Merril et al. developed a serial passage technique in mice to select phage mutants that were able to avoid removal for a prolonged period of time (62). By selecting a mutant phage, amplifying it and re-injecting it into the mice, and repeating this process 10 times, they were able to produce a phage that had a 16,000-fold higher survival rate, compared to that of normal phages. Their results showed that by using their technique and thus enhancing the

[45]

phages ability to evade the reticuloendothelial system, they achieved notably better therapeutic results. With this study, Merril *et al.* proved that rapid clearance is one of the major drawbacks of phage therapy.

8.5.2 Pharmacodynamics of Phage Therapy

The subject of pharmacodynamics is the study of the biochemical and physiological effect a drug exert on its target, and through this, on the system as a whole. This includes the mechanism of action and the relationship between drug concentration and magnitude of response (61). In terms of phage therapy, this can be broken down to a discussion of toxic *vs* therapeutic effect and concepts of accurate dosing.

The problem of toxic effect of phage therapy is believed to be less important. Partially due to the very narrow host-range of bacteriophages, and the fact that no toxic by-products are produced by phage degradation (51). Some authors claim that the release of bacterial toxins after phage lysis is a major safety concern (17,45,48,63). Abedon argues in his paper on bacteriophage pharmacology that phage therapy will be dangerous in the situation, where excessive bacterial lysis by any means may be dangerous (51). Furthermore, lessons learned from the use of phage therapy in the past and recent clinical trials, shows us that phage therapy in general produces no adverse effects (9,12,14,18,22,23,25–27,31–33,46,64).

The therapeutic effect in phage therapy with respect to pharmacodynamics is the bactericidal effect on the pathogenic bacteria. The bacteriophage mechanism of action has already been described, however, it is worth repeating the point that bacteriophages rely on chance encounters with their target in order to adsorb to the bacteria. This, the fact that bacteriophages replicate inside its host and that more than one phage can attach to the same bacteria, allows one to describe the pharmacodynamics of phage therapy as somewhat atypical in a conventional pharmacologic sense. In order to describe the circumstances to which bacteriophages at best exhibit their therapeutic effect, several concepts of killing titre, minimal inhibitory and bactericidal concentration (inundation and clearance threshold), proliferation threshold and multiplicity of infection, have been described (table 9) (ref.(51)).

The minimal inhibitory concentration is the concentration of any antibiotic pharmaceutical that is needed to prevent bacterial growth. With respect to phage therapy, this is also called the inundation threshold, which is the concentration of phages at which the rate of bacterial growth equals that of phage infection. Equally, the clearance threshold determines the concentration of phage that is needed for complete pathogen eradication (57,60).

As in the inundation and clearance threshold depends on growth of bacteria and adsorption by phages, and quantifies the amount of phages needed to clear the bacteria, it does not take into account the bacterial concentration and the factors needed for the phages to proliferate. This is taken into account in the proliferation threshold, which is defined as the concentration of bacteria needed in order for phages to increase in numbers, by means of self-amplification, with phage decay taken into account (51,59).

The common factor for all these models is that they calculate the concentration / number of phages needed in order to remove pathogenic bacteria. They differ in that some of the models take phage and bacteria replication and density into account, while others do not. Nevertheless, these models, conceived and tested in laboratory settings only, give a general rule of thumb; that bacteriophages should outnumber the bacteria by a factor of 10 in order to achieve pathogen eradication (51). Even though these models do not take into account the general diverse environment of the human body and the established truth that *in vitro* and *in vivo* observation often differ, they offer a clue for correct dosing of phage pharmaceuticals, especially in the terms of active and passive phage therapy.

8.5.3   Active *vs* Passive Phage Therapy

An important concept of utilizing bacteriophages is that they can be self-replicating pharmaceuticals, comparable e.g. to an attenuated live vaccine. As described above, laboratory studies show that in order for phage therapy to be effective one needs to achieve a sufficiently high phage to bacteria ratio. Payne and Jansen argue that many failures of phage therapy comes from an excessive reliance on the phages ability to self-replicate and to achieve a therapeutic effect by that mechanism (59). Based on this concern, the concepts of active and passive phage therapy have evolved. Although somewhat confusing terminology, the word "active" in this sense refers to reliance on phage self-amplification *in vivo* (51).

Thus, active phage therapy is the treatment protocol, where one administers one dose of phages to the patient, and lets the phages replicate, proliferate and hopefully eradicate the causative bacteria (35). In order for active phage therapy to be successful, achievement of the "proliferation threshold" is required.

The 2009 clinical trial on phage therapy of chronic otitis is an example of active phage therapy (33). The necessity of repeated dosing is warranted because the phages stopped replicating before complete pathogen eradication was achieved. In the light of Payne and Jansen's findings, this was almost obviously caused by the bacterial density falling below the proliferation threshold. Methods to overcome this problem, and thus help improve therapeutic outcome of active phage therapy, have been proposed. These include utilisation of the above described long-circulating bacteriophages and delaying therapy until bacterial concentration has reached the proliferation threshold (51,62). However, trying to overcome this hurdle may be unnecessary as the concept of passive phage therapy offers a very good alternative strategy.

Passive phage therapy is conducted by repeated administrations of bacteriophages to the patients (52). By this manner, one is able to disregard the need for phage self-replication in order to achieve sustained and sufficiently high densities. Passive phage therapy has been proposed as the gold standard for how phage therapy should be conducted (51,57,59,60). This is largely due to the high densities of phage that are required to achieve therapeutic efficacy, which are most easily accomplished through repeated administrations. An analogy to conventional pharmacology is offered by Payne and Jansen where they point to the fact that very many pharmaceutical drugs work in a dose/response relationship, and were it not for potential side-effects, the best policy would be to give the largest dose possible (60). With the relative safety and absence of side effects in phage therapy, such high doses are possible and reasonable, and best attained through passive therapy.

Table 9 - Terminology in Phage Pharmacology, according to Payne and Jansen (51,57).

Term	Definition
Minimal inhibitory concentration - MIC	A concentration at which bacterial growth is inhibited.
Inundation threshold - IT	The concentration of phages at which the rate of bacterial growth equals that of phage infection. = MIC
Clearance threshold - CT	The concentration of phages at which all bacteria are removed.
Proliferation threshold - PT	The concentration of bacteria needed in order for phages to increase in numbers, by means of self-amplification, taking phage decay into account.
Mutant selection window - MSW	The range of phage concentration at which single mutant resistant bacteria are enriched and proliferate. The lower boundary of MSW is the MIC, the upper is the MPC.
Mutant prevention concentration - MPC	Upper boundary of the MSW, dose concentration needed to eliminate the possibility for single-mutant resistant bacteria to evolve and proliferate. Multiple resistance-conferring mutations required for growth.
Multiplicity of Infection - MOI	The ratio of phages to target bacteria in a confined space
Killing titre - KT	A measure of phage density, determined in terms of the highest dilution of a phage preparation still able to kill bacteria.

In sum, in order for phage therapy to be successful, i.e., achieve complete pathogen eradication, one needs to achieve a concentration that is equal or higher than the clearance threshold. In addition, one must take into account the proliferation threshold and therefore the rate of phage decay. To "dose to cure" one therefore needs a sufficient high concentration of phages over sufficient time. In order to actually calculate the dose and time needed, one can utilise the formulas tabulated by Payne and Jansen in table 10 (ref.(60)). These, however,

[48]

have little use in a clinical setting, but offer good tools to calculate doses in a laboratory or mathematical model, which would be a crucial part of the regulatory approval efforts.

Table 10 - Formulas used to calculate phage dosing, according to Payne and Jansen (60).

Symbol	Threshold	Formula	Meaning
X_p	Proliferation threshold	$X_p = \dfrac{m(k-a)}{[bk(L-1)+ba]}$	Phage can only invade when $x(t) > X_p$
T_p	Proliferation onset time	$T_p = \dfrac{log_e[\frac{m(k-a)}{bkLx_0}]}{a}$	Optimal treatment time. Use of adjuvant antibiotic prior to T_p can be disadvantageous.
V_f	Failure density threshold	$V_f \approx \dfrac{\exp[m(T_p - T_{inoc})] - (X_p - x(T_{inoc}))m}{X_p a}$	Active therapy fails if $V_{inoc} < V_f$ for given T_{inoc}
V_i	Inundation threshold	$V_i = \dfrac{a}{b}$	Passive therapy occurs if $V_{inoc} > V_i$
V_c	Clearance threshold	$V_c \approx V_i + x(T_{inoc}) + \dfrac{log_e[x(T_{inoc})]m}{b}$	For passive therapy to fully clear bacteria $V_{inoc} > V_c$
T_h	Natural host time scale	$Tp < Th$	Determines whether active therapy is feasible

Table 11 – Legend to table 9 (60).

Symbol	Meaning
$x(t)$	Density of uninfected bacteria
x_0	Initial bacterial density at time of infection $t = 0$
V_{inoc}	Size of phage inoculum
T_{inoc}	Time of phage inoculum
a	Replication rate of bacteria
b	Adsorption constant (how rapidly a phage enters a bacteria)
k	Lysis rate
L	Burst size (number of phages released during lysis)
m	Loss rate of free phages

8.6   Major Challenges of Phage Therapy

Phage therapy is in fact facing major challenges that it needs to resolve, before it can be approved as a treatment option in Europe and North America (7,10,45,46,50,56,65). Some of these challenges were decisive in bringing about the downfall of phage therapy in the 1930s and 1940s, while others are new challenges that have emerged from the evolution of medical science and health care systems. The most commonly cited problems of phage therapy, ranging from biotechnological challenges to legal and financial issues are discussed and analysed in the sections below.

8.6.1 Phage Resistance

As antibiotic resistance is fundamental in forming the background for this thesis and many other studies on phage therapy, as well as for causing major problems and concerns in the area of infectious diseases, it will be necessary to discuss the issue of bacterial resistance to bacteriophages. In short, bacteria will develop resistance to phages very rapidly (66). However, this can be very easily circumvented by the phages ability to counter these resistance mechanisms and by smart dosing strategies.

Labrie *et al.* published in 2010 a paper on bacteriophage resistance mechanisms (67). The authors describe how bacteria evolve constantly into phage insensitive strains by means of preventing phage adsorption, preventing phage DNA entry or by cutting phage nucleic acids, and how phages adapt to this. As an example, bacteria can prevent phage adsorption by blocking its receptor, by either masking it with a protein or altering its geometric configuration. Phages overcome this changed receptor by exploiting certain genetic elements known as "diversity-generating retroelements". Simply put, these genetic elements allow the phage to substitute nucleotides in a variable region of the gene that codes for its tropism, thereby adapting to the new situation.

In their 2013 paper Ormälä and Jalasvuori questions the possibility of phage therapy suffering the same fate as antibiotics, i.e., the development of superbugs pan-resistant to bacteriophages (66). They argue that even though extensive use of bacteriophages, especially pre-determined phage cocktails, will eventually confer resistance, a new phage that is still lytic to its host-range will always be available, and that pan-phage-resistance should not be a concern. They found this when exploring global infection patterns of phages that show that environmental phages can often infect bacteria with which they lack any recent co-evolutionary history. This is because host resistance to phages is only a temporary measure, as it is disadvantageous (i.e. it loses surface structure and traits that are responsible for its virulence) for the bacteria to remain resistant to bacteriophages that are no longer present in its environment.

Ormälä and Jalasvuori argue that even though the diversity of bacteriophages and the dynamics of the bacteria-phage interaction and evolution will provide us with a supply of new phages, whenever phage resistant bacterial strains emerge, that we should be vigilant when reintroducing phage therapy, as we do not know for sure how phage resistance in hospital settings will evolve. The authors underline that care should be taken in the selection of therapeutic phages, that mass use of preformed phage cocktails should be limited and that resistance minimizing dosing strategies should be employed.

One paper that addresses this step was published by Cairns and Payne in 2008 (57). The authors modify the concept of the "mutant selection window" (MSW) to apply it to phage therapy (table 9). The MSW was originally developed as a model for dose/mutation relationship in antibiotic therapy and reflects the range of antibiotic concentrations between the minimal inhibitory concentration and the mutant prevention concentration. Dose concentrations that lie inside this "window" are selective for single mutations conferring antibiotic resistance, thus allowing for the proliferation of mutant strains. A way to close this "window" is to use combination therapy.

The authors apply this model to phage therapy, by exchanging the lower border of the MSW, the minimal inhibitory concentration, with its viral equivalent, the inundation threshold. The inundation threshold can be reached by either passive or active therapy. Passive therapy allows one to reach the inundation threshold through repeated, high dose administrations. For active therapy, on the other hand, it is essential to reach the proliferation threshold, which is dependent of bacteria concentration, in order for the phages to replicate in number and thereby reach the inundation threshold. The authors argue that even though active therapy can be achieved with a sufficiently high dose, it is not recommended due to the unpredictability of bacterial concentrations.

Moreover, Carins and Payne show that dose concentrations of phages above the inundation threshold allows for proliferation of phage-resistant, single-mutant strains. By administrating well-matched pairs of phages, by passive therapy, they were able to eradicate the population of single-mutant resistant bacteria. This is because when bacteria develops resistance through a single mutation against one of the phages used, the other phage will still be active against it, if the phage concentration is above the inundation threshold. Based on their findings they clearly recommend the use of passive phage therapy with an adapted and proven lytic cocktail of at least two phages at doses greater that the corresponding inundation threshold. Furthermore, the problem of multiple resistance is not included in the MSW, but is discussed by the authors. They argue that as multiple resistance is generally dependent on the time of the last phage administered, that passive therapy should be conducted and administered as early as possible, in order to infect all pathogenic bacteria as soon as possible.

In sum, the problem of phage resistance should be taken seriously, and careful development of treatment protocols and strategies should be developed. Bacteria will readily develop resistance against bacteriophages, but due to the vastness of the bacteriophage orders and evolutionary interaction between bacteria and phages, there will (most likely and hopefully) always be an alternative phage that will kill that bacterium. However, since this is not 100 % certain, and as we must take care to ensure that any alternative to antibiotics remains viable and does not suffer the resistance-fate, care must be taken to minimize phage resistance from day one of a theoretical phage therapy reintroduction.

8.6.2   Lack of Proper Clinical Trials and Studies

Although several encouraging case studies and reports of phage use are available, there has to date been only one randomized, double-blind, placebo-controlled clinical trial evaluating the efficacy of phage therapy (33). The lack of more systematically planned, controlled and regulated clinical trials is a decisive hindrance in reintroducing phage therapy, as stated by numerous authors (9–11,20,23,36,46,50,65,68,69). Parracho *et al.* highlighted the role and importance of regulation-abiding clinical trials in phage therapy (35).

With the pretext that randomized, double-blind, placebo-controlled clinical trials are the best way to provide vigorous and trustworthy data on the efficacy and safety of phage therapy, Parracho *et al.* details a set of factors and considerations that needs to be included and kept in mind when designing a phage therapy clinical trial. These factors are mentioned in table 12, below.

Table 12 - Factors and consideration in the design of clinical trials, according to Parracho (35).

Factor	Considerations
Study population	Should be well defined with respect to aetiology and based upon the final regulatory-approved therapeutic label, i.e. MRSA folliculitis. More details in the paragraph below this table.
Phage composition	Careful selection of lytic phages, including ensuring that they are well matched in order to increase efficacy and minimizing resistance development.
Pharmacological properties	Detailed preclinical studies of the phage preparation to determine its pharmacologic properties and to define an efficient dosing strategy.
Efficacy parameters	Primary endpoint: Patient/physician reported outcomes. Secondary endpoint: Population dynamics of aetiological agent and phages.
Safety parameters	1. Ensure the removal of debris and toxins from phage preparations. (See chapter 6.4.2) 2. Careful monitoring of immune system response, although the Herxheimer reaction has not been reported in phage therapy. (See chapter 6.6.6) 3. Ensure that only lytic phages with minimal ability for transduction are employed. (See chapter 6.6.6)
Standardisation and quality control	A well characterised phage preparation is necessary for regulatory approval, and following parameters needs thorough documentation and should be standardised: (See chapter 6.4.2) 1. Bacteriophage characterisation 2. Potency and activity of the preparation 3. Product purity 4. Stability and storage conditions 5. Control of sterility 6. Manufacturing process

Harald Brüssow argues in his 2012 paper on the challenges of phage therapy that we cannot at this time predict which diseases will be most suitable for phage therapy in a western clinical setting (46). We should therefore focus on basic research and clinical trials on obvious targets such as skin infections, eye/ear infections, and decolonisation of antibiotic resistant bacteria. By choosing this strategy, we could wait with clinical trials of more serious infections such as tuberculosis and meningitis, until the efficacy of phage therapy has been rigorously established. A key concept of double blind, placebo-controlled studies is that one group does not receive any active treatment; one can therefore hardly include patients with life-threatening and often acute diseases to such a study. The efficacy of phage therapy in such critically ill patients should therefore only be performed in the context of a comparative study, where phage therapy is measured up against the current standard treatment, after the efficacy of phage therapy in general have been unquestionably established.

Parracho *et al.* also mentions patient/physician reported outcomes as primary endpoint and population dynamics of bacteria and bacteriophages as secondary outcomes. These measurements, as well as the procedures for production, characterisation, and quality control of phage preparations should be standardised and applied to all clinical trials of phage therapy, as it would allow easy meta-analysis and interpretation across a range of studies. This would greatly contribute to allocating the evidence and proof needed to gain regulatory approval, and set an industry standard.

8.6.3   Logistical Challenges

When examining the prospect of reintroducing phage therapy, one can see that the challenges also extends to more practical problems outside the realm of scientific problems such as phage resistance and lack of proper clinical trials (50,54,56). Some of these hindrances concern the availability of therapeutic bacteriophages. As earlier described, the use of adapted and personalised phages is in a number of ways preferable to preformed phage cocktails. However, the treatment option employing adapted phages face several limitations and would need to develop strict protocols, especially concerning confirmation of diagnosis and synthesis and availability of therapeutic phages, to ensure its viability.

The identification of pathogenic bacteria is a routine laboratory procedure, employing culture or sequencing techniques. However, the concept of adapted phages includes a second step in its diagnostic scheme, namely the identification of phages that are lytic for the causative bacteria. When performed in the traditional manner, this susceptibility testing is analogous to an antibiogram, and is thus time and labour consuming (23). To alleviate this issue the maintenance of a "bank" of well-characterised, lytic bacteriophages with an determined host range, can prove as useful.

Such a "bank" could also maintain stocks of amplified bacteriophages, allowing an adapted phage cocktail to be prepared within hours of bacterial sampling (45,47,68). This, of course, anticipates the use of sequencing techniques to identify the causative bacteria, contributing to the costs of phage therapy. Furthermore, for this to be an effective and feasible treatment option, strict protocols concerning decision-making, pathogen identification, and bacteriophage "bank" maintenance need to be developed. The role of the "bank" to provide therapeutic phages in short time upon request, obliges it to continuously characterise, approve, and add phages to its collection as well as quality controlling its stocks. Although, this concept of a phage "bank" provides a decisive element in ensuring the efficacy of adapted phage therapy, it also raises several legal, regulatory, and financial questions, which may lead companies to follow the path of the less desired preformed cocktail strategy.

8.6.4 Legal Framework

Perhaps the principal yet most ambiguous problem of the prospect of phage therapy in western medicine is the regulatory and legal framework. Phage therapy in the western world first appeared and disappeared in a time where legislation governing the approval of medicinal products was quite different from what it is today. The regulatory framework imposed by the European Medicines Agency (EMA) and the Food and Drug Administration (FDA), represent comprehensive and complex legislature that is not designed for, or adapted to the idea of using natural (not modified) bacteriophages to treat bacterial infections in humans (36,50). In addition to this, the use of natural bacteriophages raises questions of Intellectual Property (IP) rights, rights that are pivotal in attracting venture capital for product development (56). This section will focus on the current legal challenges in Europe and in the USA, IP protection, as well as possible strategies to circumvent these issues.

The European Directive 2001/83/EC is the legislation governing the approval of medicinal products in the European Union and the European Economic Area. The researches behind the clinical trial on burn patients in Brussels have also published on the regulatory vacuum surrounding phage therapy in Europe, as they have faced major regulatory hurdles in gaining approval for their clinical trials (36,65,68,69). This group has also founded the non-profit organisation *Phages for Human Applications Group Europe (P.H.A.G.E)*, a group that works actively to change, clarify and adapt the European Regulatory Framework to allow for regulatory approval of bacteriophage therapeutics (23).

European regulation defines a medicinal product as "any substance presented for treating or preventing disease in human beings" (70). Interpreting this definition broadly, one can conclude that bacteriophages are medicinal products. In fact, whole animals such as leeches and larvae are approved and in use as medicinal products. As Verbeken *et al.* describes, the problems do not lie within this definition, but rather within the sub-sections of the directive that details classification and documentation requirements (36,69).

Annex 1 of the European Directive 2001/83/EC specifies the marked authorisation dossier requirements related to different pharmaceutical categories (table 13). The main issue associated with bacteriophages is that it does not fit into any of these categories, and thus impossible to fully document in an approval process.

Table 13 - Pharmaceutical categories, Annex 1 of ED 2001/83/EC (70).

Particular Medicinal Products	Advanced Therapy Medicinal Products
Biologicals	Gene therapy medicinal products
Plasma-derived	Somatic cell therapy medicinal products
Vaccines	Tissue engineered products
Radio-pharmaceuticals	
Homeopathic medicinal products	
Orphan medicinal products	
Well-established medicinal use	

Several authors cite this regulatory problem as a reason to why the larger pharmaceutical companies are refraining from developing phage pharmaceuticals (4,36,56,69). Indeed, this problem are sufficient to halt even smaller clinical trials on phage therapy, since the only way to have the phage preparations and trial approved are through local ethical committees, thus drawing large insurance fees and unnecessary safety precautions (36). The problem deepens when one takes into consideration that phage therapy is in need of a two-way regulatory approach; one for preformed phage preparations intended for marked placement, another for adapted, patient-specific phage preparations made on a case-by-case basis (69).

With this problem in mind, Verbeken *et al.* went to the European Commission to seek clarification and ask whether they would consider amending a section dedicated to phage therapy to the ED 2001/83/EC (69). They received the answer that the Commission considered the existing regulatory framework to be adequate in respect to phage therapy, without further guidance on how to interpret this.

Verbeken and his group therefore approached the EMA Innovation Task Force (ITF), with the objective of clarifying the bacteriophage classification and the documentation needed to launch clinical trials and to gain marked authorisation, in a two-way regulatory approach. In short, the ITF concluded that any pharmaceutical product utilizing natural bacteriophages will be classified as biological medicinal products, and that the documentation requirements must be evaluated on a case-by-case basis.

Although the ITF clearly states that it is feasible to gain market authorisation in Europe for bacteriophage pharmaceuticals, the route offered is impractical, long lasting, and expensive

[55]

and does not allow for easy update of phage content. Thus, following this route would allow for static phage preparations that would quickly confer resistance, and are unlikely to be profitable. The ITF offered no clear answer on how adapted, personalised phage preparations are regulated, and stated that they do not anticipate any change or amendment to the ED 2001/83/EC to be made in the foreseeable future (69).

As the legal framework in Europe can be described as bewildering at best, the situation is somewhat different in the USA. According to Harald Brüssow, one of the scientists behind the Nestle safety trial, the FDA maintains a positive attitude to phage therapy and have outlined the following profile and documentation requirements for the approval of phage therapeutics (46).

For phage preparations intended for human use, only lytic, non-transducing phages are to be used. In addition, only natural bacteriophages are acceptable, and they should not be modified to avoid immune system clearance. Each of the included phages must be characterised with a complete DNA sequence. Sterility and stability testing of the preparation as well as toxicity testing in an animal system is required. Furthermore, as the FDA considers bacteriophages as relatively low risk, not very large phase I clinical trials are needed to demonstrate the safety of the phage preparation.

Although this only serves as a rough outline of the documentation and work needed to gain approval for a medicinal product based on natural bacteriophages, it clearly shows that the FDA is willing to facilitate and adapt a regulatory process designed for bacteriophages. This stands in contrast with the above-mentioned experience with the European Commission and European Medicines Agency. The FDA have already approved several bacteriophage products for the use in the agricultural and food industry (17). The first of these products was the phage cocktail LMP-102, developed by Intralytix, that contains several phages effective against a range of pathogenic strains of *Listeria monocytogenes,* and is currently used as a food additive in the United States (57). LMP-102 was approved with the label "Generally Recognised as Safe"; a status that set precedes for the design of future phage cocktails. While these products are not subject to the more stringent requirements for products destined for human use, it shows that the FDA has recent experience in dealing with regulatory aspects of phage therapy.

Moreover, the problem of intellectual property rights is often cited as being a major factor thwarting larger pharmaceutical companies in investing in phage therapy (44,46,56,65). As bacteriophages are found in and are product of nature, patenting the phages themselves is implausible. Further, the concept of phage therapy has been around for almost a century, making it impossible for anyone to claim property rights to the technique itself. Albeit patents have been granted to the above-mentioned FDA approved phage cocktails based on cocktail character and composition, these patents have very little actual value. Because of the nature of bacteriophages, isolating a new and unique phage with the same host-range as in the patented cocktail is straightforward, effectively offering an endless assortment of free alternatives.

With the current regulatory situation in both Europe and the United States, research into phage therapy is left up to academic institutions and a handful of small, dedicated companies (12). Even though it is technically possible to develop and gain market authorisation for medicinal products based on natural bacteriophages, the existing framework is not compatible with responsible, efficient and sustainable phage therapy (65). As previously described, for phage therapy to become a true therapeutic alternative to conventional antibiotics, phages should be adapted to each individual patient and preformed phage cocktails must be updated frequently, in order to achieve maximum efficacy and minimum resistance. Under the present regulatory situation, updating a phage cocktail will require a lengthy and expensive process, effectively only allowing static cocktails to be marketed.

Clearly, a regulatory change is warranted. As Verbeken *et al.* proposed, a two-way regulatory framework dedicated to bacteriophage therapeutics, would be the ideal solution as it would clearly define and allow for personalised phage therapy, regular update of phage cocktails and a swift approval process (36,65,69). More importantly, it would create a new and feasible pharmacoeconomical paradigm, under which phage therapy may succeed.

8.6.5 Financial Concerns

The question of whether or not phage therapy can be a profitable business is the key issue for potential venture capital investors. However, this question cannot easily be answered since no phage therapy products for human use have been developed and licensed for Western world markets (56). In general, the costs of developing and attaining marked authorisation for a new drug is at least between $400 – 800 million (71). Under the current regulatory framework, it is most feasible to develop static phage cocktails, which has its obvious drawbacks in respect to conferring resistance and thereby limited usage and revenue potential.

The pharmaceutical industry has largely displayed a complete lack of interest in phage therapy. This is probably partially due to the financial uncertainty surrounding phage therapy, but also because there is a general lack of interest in developing new antibiotics in general. The ever-increasing costs of bringing a new drug to the marked have caused the pharmaceutical industry to focus their efforts on developing drugs that are intended for use over longer periods, such as blood pressure medications, thus increasing the revenue potential (4,5,71). Furthermore, with the major problem of attaining marked exclusivity and protection, it is hard to imagine that any private investor is willing to take the high investments that are required.

With this situation in mind, many authors and supporters of phage therapy have called for supranational entities such as the World Health Organisation and European Centre for Disease Control to take the lead in developing phage therapy products (46,56,65,69). The idea being that phage therapy must be considered a public necessity and should therefore be developed with public funds without financial profit as a goal. The viability of such a public endeavour is further supported by the fact that phage therapy may be cheaper than antibiotics, seen from a public health perspective (72).

Nevertheless, it is obvious that the prospect of phage under current financial and regulatory models is far from feasible, as one must rely on an international, multi-billion, non-profit project to realise it. Pirnay et al., argue that the development of a bacteriophage-specific framework will be the most efficient way to bring about a financially feasible economic model for phage therapy (65).

8.6.6   Safety Concerns and Immunological Response

Safety questions and concerns surrounding any new drug must always be thoroughly answered before the drug can be admitted to the marked. With pharmaceuticals based on bacteriophages, these safety concerns are plentiful and complex, ranging from adverse immunological reactions to gene transduction and changes in host-range.

Looking at the 90 years of experience using bacteriophages to treat humans, there are very few if any reports that the phages themselves have caused serious adverse reactions. Furthermore, we are exposed to and interact with bacteriophages our entire life and to date no illness or pathological process have been attributed to this interaction (23). This has given birth to the postulate that bacteriophages are essentially safe for humans. Although there has been a handful of safety studies that supplement the evidence of safety, there have been no studies into the cytotoxicity of phages and very few that thoroughly examine the immunological response to therapeutic phages (56).

Additionally, it is important to differentiate between the safety questions surrounding the bacteriophages themselves and the phage preparation as a whole. Past failures of phage therapy is often attributed to the crude techniques used to produce the preparations, and as shown by Merabishvili et al., this can be easily avoided by modern manufacturing methods (20).

The lack of studies on the cytotoxicity of phages can be ascribed to the general idea that phages are safe. However, as phage therapy involves applying bacteriophages in high concentrations directly into lesions where a complex inflammatory response is underway, any positive or negative modulatory effect by the bacteriophages or the preparation could affect the clinical outcome significantly (56). Gorski *et al.*, showed that bacteriophages have the ability to interact with mammalian cells expressing the β3 integrin receptor, and hence that the full extent of bacteriophage biology is not understood (8).

Bacteriophages are also capable of inducing an immune response when administered intravenously (3). One of the biggest drawbacks for the prospect for phage therapy is that repeated exposure to the same phages will trigger antibody production and dramatically decrease the efficacy of the phage preparation. Other reports suggest that bacterial remnants in crude phage lysates actually help to stimulate to immune response in a positive way, accordingly improving the clinical outcome (56). An analysis of inflammatory markers on patients undergoing phage therapy at the Phage Therapy Unit in Wroclaw, Poland, suggests that phage preparations influence and diminish the inflammatory reaction in bacterial infections (27). While there are studies focusing on the inflammatory markers and clinical outcomes, there are little evidence into the nature and extend of phage-immune system interaction, a subject that needs to be methodically scrutinised before phage therapy can be considered a serious treatment option.

Some authors have expressed the concern for transfer of virulence factors by gene transduction, as well as the possibility that some phages contain toxin-coding genes (45,63,73). This can fairly easily be overcome by careful selection of therapeutic phages and complete genome sequencing and analysis (40). Many of the safety concerns relating to phage therapy can be mitigated by sound design and Good Manufacturing Practice, to select suited bacteriophages and to remove any interfering substances from the preparations. The major issues, however, covering the precise interaction between phages, inflammatory pathways and the interaction with mammalian cells, need to be comprehensively studied in order to improve the prospect of phage therapy.

9   Discussion

The topic chosen for this thesis is thematically broad, yet narrow in the sense that relatively few previously published, comprehensive studies cover the matter. To the authors knowledge no previously published study examines the feasibility of reintroducing phage therapy to Europe and North America. Performing a feasibility study on a sparsely covered subject, with limited information on the true costs and efficacy of phage therapy, was an arduous task that required extensive studies on papers covering medicinal legislation in addition to phage therapy itself.

As a first step towards writing this review, a study protocol detailing the research design and procedure was developed. The research design, a systematic literature review, required the author to pre-determine the explicit methods through which studies were identified, data extracted and the review synthesised.

In general, the search strategy served its purpose well, and provided a comprehensive collection of studies that were evaluated against the inclusion and exclusion criteria. In hindsight, considering the low number of studies included from the electronic search, it might have been appropriate to invest even more time in fine-tuning and writing the search string in order to give a narrower and more accurate search result. The inclusion and exclusion criteria were rigorously followed, a point the author hopes helped to reduce personal bias while extracting and synthesising the data.

On the other hand, the process of coding and extracting data proved to be a time-consuming and exhausting effort, often requiring the re-reading of articles after coding had been done. The author believes he would have benefitted from investing more time in designing the coding sheet in a different manner, where more fields dedicated to specifically extracting the findings and constructs of the authors would have been prudent. Since the studies included in this project spanned a wide range of research designs, it would have been beneficial to evaluate the different order of constructs in each paper had the coding sheet been designed to do so. This would have made it easier to construct a new line of argument, based on the extracted information.

However, the author is satisfied with his coherence to the pre-determined methodology and the result as a whole. He feels that a comprehensive coverage and analysis is achieved and that this review abides by the framework of a systematic review.

9.1   The Feasibility Question

As most of the authors cited in this work mention the possible reintroduction of phage therapy and praise the potential benefits of employing bacteriophages to combat bacterial infections, it is prudent to evaluate the feasibility of such a scenario. The answer to whether or not phage therapy is feasible depends of course on how a reintroduction of phage therapy for human use is defined. To create an extensive analysis, two different setups for reintroduction will be discussed in the paragraphs below. The two different scenarios are; (i) phage therapy modelled after current practice in Georgia, and (ii) phage therapy modelled after current practice in Poland.

A reintroduction of phage therapy modelled after current use in Georgia will involve a general introduction of phage therapeutics active against a wide spectrum of bacterial infections. In Georgia, phage therapy is available as phage cocktails sold over the counter and as prescribed and personalised therapy (14,24). The lytic spectra of the cocktails are evaluated every six months and, if necessary, updated with new phages. Prescribed phage therapy, involves the identification of the patients pathogenic bacteria and selection of one or more phages accordingly. Phage therapy according to the Georgian model can serve as a first line treatment option and not only as a last resort after antibiotic treatment has failed. As this mode of phage therapy is dynamic, where one routinely changes the phages used and employing the concept of a phage bank, it can easily be adapted in response to emerging resistance patterns. Therefore, this type of phage therapy is suitable for creating a long-term, sensible, and viable treatment alternative to conventional antibiotic, covering a wide range of infections (68).

However, this approach is not without its disadvantages. Under the current regulatory regime in Europe and North America, phage therapy by this model stands no chance. As Verbeken and Pirnay have stated, a distinct set of regulations allowing for easy update of phage cocktails and selection of phages for personalised therapy are needed if this is to be practically and economically viable (65,69). The cost of developing and updating phage cocktails associated with current regulations cannot be defended by any commercial entity under the lack of market protection. As this model of phage therapy involves products for marked placement, it is not up to academic institutions alone to drive its development. As the commercial sector will be vital in this effort, a possible solution, in addition to regulatory change, can be public-private investments and extended marked exclusivity and rights. Nevertheless, regardless of marked incentives and public money invested, this model of phage therapy can only be developed as a sustainable alternative to antibiotics under new bacteriophage-specific regulations.

In Poland, phage therapy is currently practiced as an experimental treatment for antibiotic resistant infections (25). That is, all patients receive personalised therapy where phages handpicked for the identified causative bacteria are administered. This method of personalised medicine requires the maintenance of a phage bank, and developed infrastructure for rapid and precise pathogen identification. Although not proven by means of randomised clinical trials, results indicate that this mode of phage therapy can achieve pathogen eradication in 20 % of patients. This model of phage therapy is currently employed as a last resort measure, when antibiotic treatment has failed.

Reintroducing phage therapy in the manner currently employed in Poland, can offer hope for some patients, but does not represent a true alternative to antibiotics, as it would only be employed as a second or last line treatment option, thereby still depending on antibiotics for the vast majority of bacterial infections. In order for this phage therapy option to be considered as a sustainable treatment option and alternative, it would need to be used as a first line treatment. This will require a sound and efficient, yet costly infrastructure in respect to diagnosis, pathogen identification, and preparation of therapeutic phages. Even though this is a question of money and expertise, which can be provided through public funds and academic institutions, there is still a void in the regulatory framework on personalised phage therapy.

A widespread, continued use of personalised phage therapy under an experimental regulatory umbrella, as in Poland, is neither desirable nor feasible for the duration. It is therefore vital that regulations detailing the operations of a phage bank and preparation of personalised phage solutions are formulated. Such regulations should provide a standardised method for gaining approval for individual phages, which can then be amplified and stored until required for use. Sound regulations in this field could also make phage banks profitable, thereby creating incentive for private investors to invest in phage therapy and research.

Both the above-mentioned models of phage therapy are hampered by the regulatory situation in the western world. They do also share another problem; the uncertainty of efficacy of phage therapy. Even though some reports suggest that phage therapy have been successful in 80-90 % of patients, the real figure is probably much lower and probably in the range of 20 % (18,22,25,33). The fact being, that the blatant lack of randomised, clinical trials leaves researchers, authors and policy-makers with important unanswered questions of phage therapy efficacy. If public funds were to be used in large-scale development of phage therapy, sound evidence regarding its efficacy will first need to be established. Additionally, it is likely that the decision-makers, who control the money, will be sceptical to invest into a treatment option that may cure as few as 20 % of the patients.

Both the Georgian and Polish models of phage therapy suffer under the current medicinal regulations, pharmacoeconomic environment, and its own lack of clinical trials. Under existing regulatory framework, neither of these options are to be considered as feasible as a therapeutic alternative to antibiotics. While regulatory change would alleviate this situation greatly, by attracting investors and enable proper clinical trials, this author finds it unlikely to

[62]

believe that new regulations dedicated and tailored for phage therapy will soon become a reality.

10 Conclusion

As discussed in previous chapters, that challenges for a possible reintroduction of phage therapy are many. Firstly, although anecdotal evidence from 90 years of use hints to a degree of safety and efficacy, this is insufficient to serve as a building block on the way to market authorisation. Secondly, the medicinal legislation in Europe and North America does not allow for a meaningful, responsible, efficient, and sustainable use of therapeutic bacteriophages. Thirdly, and lastly, due to the lack of interest from the pharmaceutical industry there is a blatant lack of money to finance further studies and clinical trials, leaving the research mostly with academic institutions.

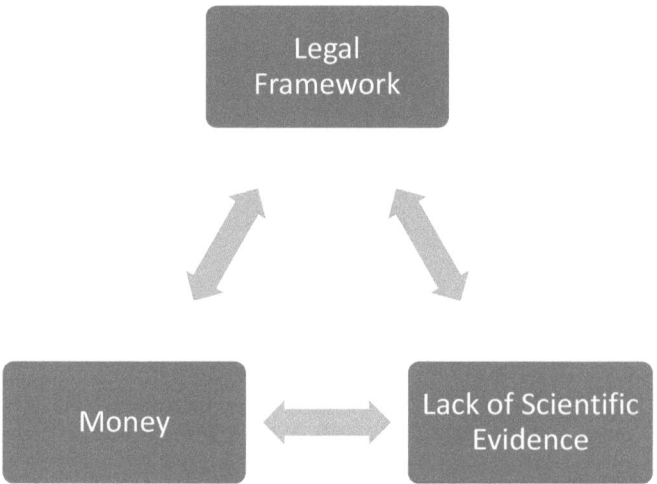

Figure 8 . Main hurdles for the reintroduction of phage therapy.

This troika of problems are both interconnected and dependent on each other, and one can greatly improve the prospect of phage therapy reintroduction, if one manages to break the chain at any point (Fig. 9). That is, if someone chose to invest in a project designed to create a base of solid evidence concerning phage therapy, the regulatory change might be easier to bring about, and vice versa. Hence, a change in the positive direction at any of these points may bring about the others and pave the way for phage therapy.

A Belgian bacteriophage research group believes that the best point of attack on this troika is the legal framework. They argue that a regulatory framework designed for phage therapy is the best way to create a foundation and milieu that attracts investors and where clinical trials can be undertaken. This would indeed be the most desirable method, as it would not only create a platform for phage therapy but also a radical change to the pharmacoeconomic attitude towards developing drugs for antimicrobial use.

However, this author does not share the Belgian scientists´ optimism in believing in a regulatory change. With the current political systems in Europe and North America, changing legislations is a time consuming process subject to numerous committees and political procedures. Without a proper and supportive legal setting, it is also highly unlikely that investors will invest the amounts needed to conduct the research required. Therefore, the prospect of phage therapy remains obscure, and is likely to stay so in the near future.

Moreover, some scientists have used the argument that one should take the lessons learned from phage therapy, and use this knowledge to develop novel treatment modalities (5,7,17,30,45,48,50,74). The most obvious examples of this are the use of phage lysins, and engineered bacteriophages. Phage lysins have been shown to have a great potential, both as a mono-drug and in conjunction with antibiotics. To this date, there are no reports of resistance to lysins, although they may arise, this new class of enzybiotics shows promise and is facing a much brighter prospect concerning regulatory hindrances and finances. The notion of engineering bacteriophages ranges from making minor alterations in the genome of the phage, to constructing nanoparticles that uses similar targeting techniques as bacteriophages to deliver lysins or other bactericidal compounds directly to its target. If altered sufficiently, and designed from scratch these engineered phages / nanoparticles are covered by existing regulation, and offer a much better chance of yielding a feasible product.

In the end, products derived from the knowledge on bacteriophages stand a much better chance to provide an alternative to antibiotics, not necessarily due to superior efficacy or lesser side effects, but due to the legal, financial, and scientific demands of our society. These derived products conform to our demands and framework in a completely different way than natural bacteriophages do. As bringing about new classes of antibiotics and other alternatives is overdue with several decades, it is the opinion of this author that research into products derived from bacteriophages should be prioritized above research into natural bacteriophages.

Consequently, I cannot consider phage therapy based on natural bacteriophages to be a feasible alternative to antibiotics under the current situation, they should, however, be hailed for providing invaluable knowledge about other possible treatment options that can provide a solution to the antibiotic resistance crisis.

11 Bibliography

1. Khardori N. Antibiotics--past, present, and future. Med Clin North Am. 2006;90:1049–76.

2. Livermore DM. The need for new antibiotics. Clin Microbiol Infect. 2004;10:1–9.

3. Taylor PW, Stapelton PD, Paul LJ. New ways to treat bacterial infections. Drugs Discov Today. 2002;7:1086 – 1091.

4. Projan SJ. Why is big Pharma getting out of antibacterial drug discovery? Curr Opin Microbiol. 2003 6:427–30.

5. Powers JH. Antimicrobial drug development--the past, the present, and the future. Clin Microbiol Infect. 2004;10:23–31.

6. Fischbach M, Walsh C. Antibiotics for emerging pathogens. Science. 2009;325:1089–93.

7. Fernebro J. Fighting bacterial infections-future treatment options. Drug Resist Updat. 2011;14:125–39.

8. Gorski A, Dabrowska K, Switala-Jele K, Nowaczyk M, Weber-Dabrowska B, Baratynski J, et al. New insights into the possible role of bacteriophages in host defense and disease. Med Immunol. 2003;2.

9. Abedon ST, Kuhl SJ, Blasdel BG, Kutter EM. Phage treatment of human infections. Bacteriophage. 2011;1:66–85.

10. Mattey M, Spencer J. Bacteriophage therapy--cooked goose or phoenix rising? Curr Opin Biotechnol. 2008;19:608–12.

11. Sulakvelidze A, Alavidze Z. Bacteriophage Therapy. Antimicrob Agents Chemother. 2001;45:649–59.

12. Deresinski S. Bacteriophage therapy: exploiting smaller fleas. Clin Infect Dis. 2009 15;48:1096–101.

13. Abedon ST, Thomas-Abedon C, Thomas A, Mazure H. Bacteriophage prehistory: Is or is not Hankin, 1896, a phage reference? Bacteriophage. 2011;1:174–8.

14. Chanishvili N. Phage therapy--history from Twort and d'Herelle through Soviet experience to current approaches. Adv Virus Res. 1st ed. Elsevier Inc.; 2012;83:3–40.

15. Twort F. An investigation on the nature of ultra-microscopic viruses. Lancet. 1915;186:1241–3.

16. D'Herelle F. On an invisible microbe antagonistic toward dysenteric bacilli. Comptes Rendus Acad des Sci. 1917;165:373–5.

17. Lu TK, Koeris MS. The next generation of bacteriophage therapy. Curr Opin Microbiol. 2011;14:524–31.

18.   Alisky J, Iczkowski K, Rapoport A, Troitsky N. Bacteriophages show promise as antimicrobial agents. J Infect. 1998;36:5–15.

19.   Barrow P a, Soothill JS. Bacteriophage therapy and prophylaxis: rediscovery and renewed assessment of potential. Trends Microbiol. 1997;5:268–71.

20.   Merabishvili M, Pirnay J-P, Verbeken G, Chanishvili N, Tediashvili M, Lashkhi N, et al. Quality-controlled small-scale production of a well-defined bacteriophage cocktail for use in human clinical trials. PLoS One. 2009;4:e4944.

21.   Eaton M, Bayne-Jones S. Bacteriophage Therapy. J Am Med Assoc. 1934;8:1769.

22.   Weber-Dąbrowska B, Mulczyk M, Górski A. Bacteriophage therapy of bacterial infections: an update of our institute's experience. Arch Immunol Ther Exp (Warsz). 2000;48:547–51.

23.   Kutter E, De Vos D, Gvasalia G, Alavidze Z, Gogokhia L, Kuhl S, et al. Phage therapy in clinical practice: treatment of human infections. Curr Pharm Biotechnol. 2010;11:69–86.

24.   Chanishvili N. A Literature Review of the Practical Application of Bacteriophage Research. 1st ed. Sharp R, editor. Tbilisi: Eliava Institute; 2009.

25.   Międzybrodzki R, Borysowski J, Weber-Dąbrowska B, Fortuna W, Letkiewicz S, Szufnarowski K, et al. Clinical aspects of phage therapy. Adv Virus Res. 2012;83:73–121.

26.   Borysowski J, Górski A. Is phage therapy acceptable in the immunocompromised host? Int J Infect Dis. 2008;12:466–71.

27.   Miedzybrodzki R, Fortuna W, Weber-Dabrowska B, Górski A. A retrospective analysis of changes in inflammatory markers in patients treated with bacterial viruses. Clin Exp Med. 2009;9:303–12.

28.   Weber-Dabrowska B, Zimecki M, Kruzel M, Kochanowska I, Lusiak-Szelachowska M. Alternative therapies in antibiotic-resistant infection. Adv Med Sci. 2006;51:242–4.

29.   Slopek S, Weber-Dabrowska B, Dabrowski M, Kucharewicz-Krukowska A. Results of bacteriophage treatment of suppurative bacterial infections in the years 1981-1986. Arch Immunol Ther Exp (Warsz). 1987;35:569–83.

30.   O'Flaherty S, Ross RP, Coffey A. Bacteriophage and their lysins for elimination of infectious bacteria. FEMS Microbiol Rev. 2009;33:801–19.

31.   Bruttin A, Brüssow H. Human volunteers receiving Escherichia coli phage T4 orally: a safety test of phage therapy. Antimicrob Agents Chemother. 2005;49:2874–8.

32.   Sarker SA, McCallin S, Barretto C, Berger B, Pittet A-C, Sultana S, et al. Oral T4-like phage cocktail application to healthy adult volunteers from Bangladesh. Virology. 2012;434:222–32.

33.   Wright a, Hawkins CH, Anggård EE, Harper DR. A controlled clinical trial of a therapeutic bacteriophage preparation in chronic otitis due to antibiotic-resistant

Pseudomonas aeruginosa; a preliminary report of efficacy. Clin Otolaryngol. 2009;34:349–57.

34. Soothill J, Hawkins C, Anggar E, Harper D. Therapeutic use of bacteriophages. Lancet Infect Dis. 2004;4:544–5.

35. Parracho HM, Burrowes BH, Enright MC, McConville ML, Harper DR. The role of regulated clinical trials in the development of bacteriophage therapeutics. J Mol Genet Med. 2012;6:279–86.

36. Verbeken G, De Vos D, Vaneechoutte M, Merabishvili M, Zizi M, Pirnay J-P. European regulatory conundrum of phage therapy. Future Microbiol. 2007;2:485–91.

37. Forterre P. The origin of viruses and their possible roles in major evolutionary transitions. Virus Res. 2006;117:5–16.

38. Ackermann H. Bacteriophage taxonomy. Microbiol Aust. 2011;32:90–4.

39. Ackermann H. Bacteriophage observations and evolution. Res Microbiol. 2003;154:245–51.

40. Matsuzaki S, Rashel M, Uchiyama J, Sakurai S, Ujihara T, Kuroda M, et al. Bacteriophage therapy: a revitalized therapy against bacterial infectious diseases. J Infect Chemother. 2005;11:211–9.

41. Walker J. Bacteriophages. 1st ed. Clokie MRJ, Kropinski AM, editors. Totowa, NJ: Humana Press; 2009.

42. Skurnik M, Strauch E. Phage therapy: facts and fiction. Int J Med Microbiol. 2006;296:5–14.

43. Filippov A a, Sergueev K V, Nikolich MP. Can phage effectively treat multidrug-resistant plague? Bacteriophage. 2012;2:186–9.

44. Clark JR, March JB. Bacteriophages and biotechnology: vaccines, gene therapy and antibacterials. Trends Biotechnol. 2006;24:212–8.

45. Skurnik M, Pajunen M, Kiljunen S. Biotechnological challenges of phage therapy. Biotechnol Lett. 2007;29:995–1003.

46. Brüssow H. What is needed for phage therapy to become a reality in Western medicine? Virology. 2012;434:138–42.

47. Gill JJ, Hyman P. Phage choice, isolation, and preparation for phage therapy. Curr Pharm Biotechnol. 2010;11:2–14.

48. Goodridge LD. Designing phage therapeutics. Curr Pharm Biotechnol. 2010;11:15–27.

49. Golshahi L, Seed KD, Dennis JJ, Finlay WH. Toward modern inhalational bacteriophage therapy: nebulization of bacteriophages of Burkholderia cepacia complex. J Aerosol Med Pulm Drug Deliv. 2008;21:351–60.

[68]

50. Chan BK, Abedon ST, Loc-Carrillo C. Phage cocktails and the future of phage therapy. Future Microbiol. 2013;8:769–83.

51. Abedon ST, Thomas-Abedon C. Phage therapy pharmacology. Curr Pharm Biotechnol. 2010;11:28–47.

52. Ryan EM, Gorman SP, Donnelly RF, Gilmore BF. Recent advances in bacteriophage therapy: how delivery routes, formulation, concentration and timing influence the success of phage therapy. J Pharm Pharmacol. 2011;63:1253–64.

53. Dabrowska K, Switała-Jelen K, Opolski A, Weber-Dabrowska B, Gorski A. Bacteriophage penetration in vertebrates. J Appl Microbiol. 2005;98:7–13.

54. Maura D, Debarbieux L. Bacteriophages as twenty-first century antibacterial tools for food and medicine. Appl Microbiol Biotechnol. 2011;90:851–9.

55. Westwater C, Kasman L. Use of genetically engineered phage to deliver antimicrobial agents to bacteria: an alternative therapy for treatment of bacterial infections. Antimicrob Agents Chemother. 2003;47:1301–7.

56. Henein A. What are the limitations on the wider therapeutic use of phage? Bacteriophage. 2013;3:1–7.

57. Cairns BJ, Payne RJH. Bacteriophage therapy and the mutant selection window. Antimicrob Agents Chemother. 2008;52:4344–50.

58. Cairns BJ, Timms AR, Jansen V a a, Connerton IF, Payne RJH. Quantitative models of in vitro bacteriophage-host dynamics and their application to phage therapy. PLoS Pathog. 2009;5:e1000253.

59. Payne RJ, Phil D, Jansen VA. Phage therapy: the peculiar kinetics of self-replicating pharmaceuticals. Clin Pharmacol Ther. 2000;68:225–30.

60. Payne RJH, Jansen V a a. Pharmacokinetic principles of bacteriophage therapy. Clin Pharmacokinet. 2003;42:315–25.

61. Harvey R, Champe P. Lippincott's Illustrated Reviews: Pharmacology, 4th Edition. 4th ed. Medicine & Science in Sports & Exercise. Philadelphia: Lippincott Williams & Wilkins; 2008.

62. Merril CR, Biswas B, Carlton R, Jensen NC, Creed GJ, Zullo S, et al. Long-circulating bacteriophage as antibacterial agents. Proc Natl Acad Sci U S A. 1996 16;93:3188–92.

63. Martínez J, Baquero F. Interactions among strategies associated with bacterial infection: pathogenicity, epidemicity, and antibiotic resistance. Clin Microbiol Rev. 2002;15:647–79.

64. Levin B, Bull J. Phage therapy revisited: the population biology of a bacterial infection and its treatment with bacteriophage and antibiotics. Am Nat. 1996;147:881–98.

65. Pirnay J-P, Verbeken G, Rose T, Jennes S, Zizi M, Huys I, et al. Introducing yesterday's phage therapy in today's medicine. Future Virol. 2012;7:379–90.

66. Ormälä A-M, Jalasvuori M. Phage therapy: Should bacterial resistance to phages be a concern, even in the long run? Bacteriophage. 2013;3:e24219.

67. Labrie SJ, Samson JE, Moineau S. Bacteriophage resistance mechanisms. Nat Rev Microbiol. 2010;8:317–27.

68. Pirnay J-P, De Vos D, Verbeken G, Merabishvili M, Chanishvili N, Vaneechoutte M, et al. The phage therapy paradigm: prêt-à-porter or sur-mesure? Pharm Res. 2011;28:934–7.

69. Verbeken G, Pirnay J-P, De Vos D, Jennes S, Zizi M, Lavigne R, et al. Optimizing the European regulatory framework for sustainable bacteriophage therapy in human medicine. Arch Immunol Ther Exp (Warsz). 2012;60:161–72.

70. European Directive 2001/83/EC - Community code relating to medicinal products for human use. The European Union; 2001.

71. DiMasi J a, Hansen RW, Grabowski HG. The price of innovation: new estimates of drug development costs. J Health Econ. 2003;22:151–85.

72. Miedzybrodzki R, Fortuna W, Weber-Dabrowska B, Górski A. Phage therapy of staphylococcal infections (including MRSA) may be less expensive than antibiotic treatment. Postepy Hig Med Dosw (Online). 2007;61:461–5.

73. Górski A, Weber-Dabrowska B. The potential role of endogenous bacteriophages in controlling invading pathogens. Cell Mol Life Sci. 2005;62:511–9.

74. Lu TK, Collins JJ. Engineered bacteriophage targeting gene networks as adjuvants for antibiotic therapy. Proc Natl Acad Sci U S A. 2009;106:4629–34.

12 Appendix

12.1 Coding Sheet

<u>Revised Final Coding Sheet 18.10.13</u>

(Adapted BEME coding sheet)

1. Reference information:

- **Reference number in Mendeley:** _____

- **Date extracted (e) and date coded (c): e:_____   c:_____**

- **Publication type:**

  □ Book   □ Journal Article

                                                       o   Review

                                                       o   original article

                                                       o   letter/commentary

  □ Non-peer reviewed article   □ Conference paper

  □ Official publication   □ Thesis

  □ Other: □ Patent application,

                                                  □ Pharmacopoieas

- **Citation information:**

  Author (s):

  Title:

  Publication (Journal name):

  Year: **Volume:**   **Issue:**   **Pages**:

- **Search method:**

  □ Electronic search   □ Personal recommendation

  □ Hand search   □ Grey literature

  □ Other:

2. **Evaluation of Methods:**

- **Research design:** (tick all that apply)

  Non-comparative studies:

  □ Audit   □ Expert opinion   □ Report

  □ Observation   □ Case-series   □ Historical

Comparative studies:	**Single group studies**	**Cohort study:**
□ Cross Sectional	□ Before & after studies	□ Prospective
□ Case control	□ Time series	□ Retrospective

  Trails:

  □ Randomized   □ controlled   □ double blinded

  □ Not randomized   □ uncontrolled □ not / single blinded

  □ Phase I   □ Phase II   □ Phase III

  Review:

  □ Review – Details: □ Cites evidence w/data   □ Conceptual

                                      □ Descriptive   □ Commentary

  □ Meta – analysis – Details:

- **Data collection methods:** (tick all that apply)

  □ Interview   □ Observation   □ Opinion

  □ Patient outcomes   □ Data from simulator/simulation

  □ Literature search   □ Other:

3. **Context:**
   - **Number of subjects: (if applicable)**
   - **Intervention:**
   - **Location of study:**
   - **Outcome:**
   - **Field of study relevant to this thesis:**

   □ Virology   □ Clinical application   □ Immunology

   □ Antibiotic resistance   □ Legal framework   □ Clinical trail

   □ Other: □ History   □ Pharmacology

4. **Aim of study:**
   - **Objective /aim / purpose**   □ Stated   □ Not available
     - Details:

   - **Based on relevant literature**   □ Stated   □ Not available
     - Specify whether the author demonstrated awareness of the literature:

5. **Does the publication help to answer any of the following questions:**

   □ How were bacteriophages discovered and studied?

   □ What are the bacteriophage molecular structure, classification and mechanism of action?

   □ What are the possible medicinal applications of bacteriophages?

   □ Which are documented uses and/or clinical trails of bacteriophages?

   □ How have bacteriophages been applied clinically,

   - with respect to confirmation of diagnosis,
   - synthesis of therapeutic bacteriophages or
   - administration to patient?

   □ How does the human body's immune system respond to bacteriophages?

   □ How feasible is bacteriophage therapy?

   □ How is the European regulatory framework in respect to bacteriophage therapy in human medicine?

[73]

6. **Author´s findings:**

7. **Strength of findings:**
   ☐ No clear results can be drawn. Not significant

   ☐ Results ambiguous, but there appears to be a trend

   ☐ Conclusions can probably be based on the results

   ☐ Results are clear and very likely to be true. Results are unequivocal

   ☐ No original data (review publication)

8. **Notes:**

12.2 Statistics of Cited Studies

Table 14 - Types of studies cited

Study Design	Number Cited
Clinical Trial	4
Case reports	6
Laboratory models and studies	11
Books	3
Literature Reviews	49
Laws	1
Total	**74**

Table 15 - Thematic groups and number of studies allocated.

Thematic Group	Number of Studies Allocated (One study can be allocated to more than one group)
Antibiotic resistance	7
Financial concerns of drug development	5
History of phage therapy	14
Immune system response to phages	12
Legal challenges to phage therapy	15
Other uses of bacteriophages	6
Pharmacology of bacteriophages	8
Safety concerns of phage therapy	11
Virology of bacteriophages	20

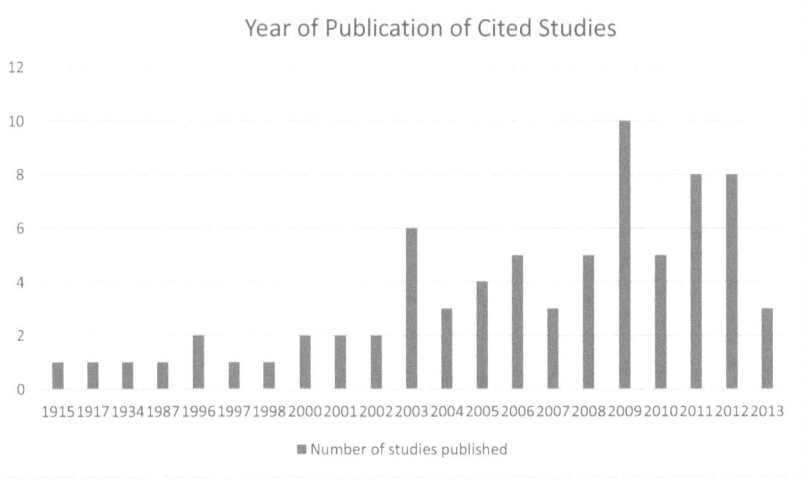

Figure 9 - Year of Publication of Cited Studies

12.3 List of Tables and Figures

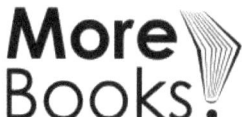
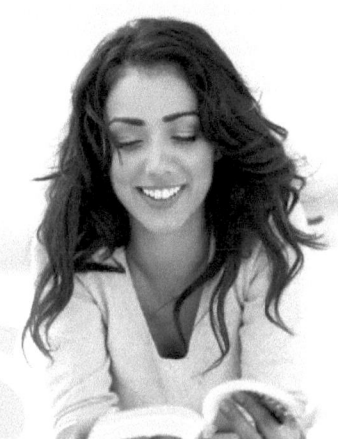

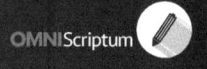

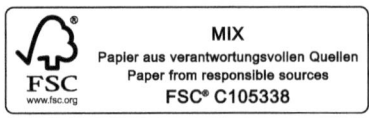
Printed by Books on Demand GmbH, Norderstedt / Germany